When it Hurts to Care
Clergy Working with Crisis

By Jill Hendron

When it Hurts to Care

Clergy Working with Crisis

By Jill Hendron

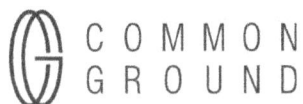

COMMON GROUND

First published in 2022
as part of the *Religion in Society* Book Imprint
doi: 10.18848/978-1-86335-264-2/CGP (Full Book)

Common Ground Research Networks
2001 South First Street, Suite 202
University of Illinois Research Park
Champaign, IL
61820

Library of Congress Cataloging-in-Publication Data

Names: Hendron, Jill, author.
Title: *When it hurts to care: Clergy Working with Crisis* / by Jill Hendron
Description: Champaign, IL: Common Ground Research Networks, 2021. |
    Includes bibliographical references. | Summary: "This book explores the
    emotional, physical, and spiritual toll that affects those in the caring
    professions. The immediate subject matter focus on clergy is relevant to
    a wide range of professions who support others as the issue of the cost
    of caring has become even more salient due to the ongoing pandemic. This
    book is also an essential text book for clergy training and for other
    caring professions. The world has changed significantly since the
    pandemic and the wider concept of wellness and support have gained a
    wider audience as well"-- Provided by publisher.
Identifiers: LCCN 2021037999 (print) | LCCN 2021038000 (ebook) | ISBN
    9780949313676 (hardback) | ISBN 9781863352635 (paperback) | ISBN
    9781863352642 (adobe pdf)
Subjects: LCSH: Pastoral care. | Psychic trauma--Religious
    aspects--Christianity. | Crisis management--Religious
    aspects--Christianity. | Caring--Religious aspects--Christianity.
Classification: LCC BV4012 .H435 2021 (print) | LCC BV4012 (ebook) | DDC
    253.5/2--dc23
LC record available at https://lccn.loc.gov/2021037999
LC ebook record available at https://lccn.loc.gov/202103800

Table of Contents

Acknowlegment

Firstly, many thanks go to everyone at Common Ground Research Networks for nurturing this book to completion. To all those who have ever taken the time to either devise or respond to a research study, without you, books such as this would not be possible. There are many people and who both professionally and personally have contributed indirectly to this book through their support and encouragement. To them all and especially my children and their families I thank you. Finally, my unending thanks to Paul who will not like the direct mention, but it needs said as this book would never have happened without you!

Chapter 1

Introduction

"There is a cost to caring. Professionals who listen to clients' stories of fear, pain and suffering may feel similar fear, pain and suffering because they care" (Figley, 1995, p1).

The aim of this book is to extend the conversation around challenging aspects of the pastoral ministry. There have been numerous valuable publications on the more generic aspects of ministerial stress but this specific aspect has not yet been adequately explored. As such the focus of this book will move beyond the general and will look more specifically at the challenges and costs of working with those individuals and communities who have experienced trauma and crisis.

At times the world can be a challenging place and perhaps none more so that than during the current period of the Covid 19 pandemic which is currently spreading distress, fear and uncertainty across the globe. Whilst much of this book was written in a pre-Covid 19 world, the final revisions were being added as the pandemic stuck and as such the evolving crisis situation and the appearance of faith leaders on media broadcasts describing the human toll that the virus is exacting has made the extension of this conversation even more essential to building an understanding of the fundamental challenges faced when providing pastoral care.

This opening chapter sets the scene for the book and hopefully affords readers a foretaste of what is to follow by discussing briefly the background to the book and the context in which it is placed.

My interest in the challenges and costs of working with those who have experienced trauma arose from two important sources. Firstly, from over twenty years' personal experience working as a bereavement counsellor. This work clearly demonstrated that emotional care for others can and does leave an imprint and demands a cost from those who provide much-needed support. Indeed, those who provide emotional care can perhaps unknowingly place themselves at risk of personal and professional costs simply through caring.

Secondly, anecdotal evidence from clergy suggested there were more challenges taking place within their professional and personal lives than were immediately evident. It is important to state at this juncture that whilst there is an expanding understanding of stress in the ministry, anecdotal evidence suggests something more complex is occurring. Therefore, the current understanding of general stress and occupational burnout do not necessarily provide an adequate analysis of what appears to be taking place within the clergy setting.

The amalgamation of these two factors resulted in the doctoral study on which this book is grounded. The findings that emerged from this study opened avenues that I had not completely foreseen and enabled me to embark on various speaking and presenting engagements both within the academic sphere and within ministerial domains; engaging with clergy in training, serving clergy and those already retired. Whilst the context of my doctoral study was Ireland, encounters with clergy from different parts of the globe confirmed that sadly this was not merely an issue confined to Irish clergy or in one specific theological denomination, nor was it restricted to Ireland's specific form of troubles related trauma. Instead, there appears to be a troublesome issue around working with trauma that is alive and well within the pastoral ministry of many clergy who serve within a variety of denominations and throughout numerous geographical locations.

The successful completion of my doctoral thesis and the issues it uncovered led inevitably to the development of this book as it was seen as a means of broadening the debate and providing a more widely available exploration of a topic that was long overdue. Additionally, for any exploration of this subject area to have the credibility and significance it merits, it is imperative the topic be dealt with within the robust framework of academic research, published discussions and underpinning anecdotal evidence. Therefore, whilst every attempt has been made to present the discussion in a manner that is palatable to a wide audience, there will be a consistent return to literature that validates and supports the debate.

Through advancing an understanding of the experiences of those who, within the pastoral ministry, provide care and compassion for victims and survivors of trauma this book is intended for several audiences. Firstly, it will naturally be beneficial for those who personally undertake this work within their pastoral role. Secondly, it will be of value to those who are in any way responsible for the care and support of these individuals, the contents will be valuable in informing training, preparation and support of clergy when connecting with those who have experienced trauma and crisis.

There is a complex story to be told within this book and one that must be unpacked copiously to be fully understood. Much consideration has been given to its composition and progression to ensure that the story being told is logical and robust and encompasses both theoretical concepts and personal experiences. It is my hope that those who read it will find its contents to be of value for themselves, their ministry and for the hurting individuals and communities that they care for.

Chapter 2

Setting the Scene: Clergy & Crisis

Increasingly those who have chosen the vocational route of clergy life have perhaps without realising it embarked upon a hazardous journey, (Hendron et al., 2012). Undoubtedly, it is recognised that the ministry presents personal and professional challenges and that clergy, like other caring professionals, are especially vulnerable to occupational stress (Francis et al., 2009) and it has been suggested that the resulting consequence for a parish may be a cleric who is unable to assist those who require support for coping with stressors due to the fact they are unable to cope with the challenges of their own ministry (Terry & Cunningham, 2020).

The emergence of such recognition and the development of a robust body of knowledge around the wider concept of clergy occupational stress should be greatly welcomed. However, the requirements of the pastoral ministry involve integration and support for both individuals and communities and perhaps never more so than at times of crisis. Therefore, a much more specific understanding of the impact of these interactions is needed over and above understanding general stress reactions or occupational burnout.

The past few decades have seen recognition emerge that those who provide care and support for individuals, families and communities who have experienced crisis are themselves at risk of experiencing an adverse impact, (Sabo, 2006). However, despite it being widely accepted that clergy are often at the forefront of helping others with crisis in their lives (Leavey et al., 2007; Leavey, 2008; Jankowski et al., 2011) and as such spend long hours in stressful and emotionally demanding situations that can have an exacting toll (Darling et al., 2004), empirical exploration and everyday acknowledgement of the impact upon clergy when working with trauma has been scarce and only a few academic studies have emerged which begin to offer some insights.

As with many aspects of life academic theories emerge in attempts to help us capture and hopefully understand these experiences. The growing recognition that there is a cost to caring has led to the emergence of several such theories or conceptualisations that attempt to capture either the negative or positive impact of working vicariously with trauma. These include the concepts of Secondary Traumatic Stress, also referred to as Compassion Fatigue (Figley, 1995), and Vicarious Traumatisation (McCann & Pearlman, 1990a), all of which will be discussed in detail in due course.

In an attempt to understand these issues within a wide range of contexts, academic interest has examined a range of divers professions which include inter alia; mental health professionals (Cranfield, 2005; Versola-Russo, 2007; Way et al., 2007; Devilly et al., 2009; Harrison & Westwood, 2009); social workers (Lekkos, 2008; Ying, 2009); nursing staff (Maytum et al., 2004; Lev-Wiesel et al., 2009);

teachers (Lucas, 2008); counsellors (Jenkins & Baird, 2002; Benoit et al., 2007; Sommer, 2008); the judicial sector (Jaffe et al., 2006; Chamberlain & Miller, 2009).

Seeking to understand what occurs within our professional lives is no new thing. We constantly strive to make sense of what we experience and this knowledge should add to our understanding of how to care for ourselves and protect the wellbeing of others and ourselves. Such is the case with the emergence of these concepts as each has in its own way added another layer of understanding and as Figley (1995) contended, each has provided us with a terminology which solely captured the impact of working with human crisis and trauma as opposed to the more general stress associated with the workplace. If we are accepting that there is an impact from caring, especially during times of crisis, then naturally we need to understand how the role of the pastoral ministry places individual clergy at the centre of these storms. Therefore, before this book moves forward to unpack the impact of caring within the ministry it will take some time to examine the elements of the pastoral ministry that perhaps place clergy at the greatest risk.

Pastoral care is recognised as a fundamental part of the clergy role (Weaver et al., 2003; Farrell & Goebert, 2008; Leavey, 2008). Gillman et al. (1996.p16) exploring pastoral care state, '*Any pastoral intervention assumes a caring presence, a compassionate heart, and continued active listening*'. Additionally, clergy are frequently accessed during times of trauma and crisis (Stanford & McAlister, 2008). Some clergy have anecdotally suggested that they are not at risk from the impact of emotionally caring as they do not provide specific counselling support to their parishioners and therefore such discussions are not relevant to them. However, being involved in a 'formal' counselling relationship is not essential to experiencing vicarious impact but instead exposure to and interaction with human pain and suffering is essentially the trigger. Lee (1980) provides a useful distinction in the differences between pastoral care and pastoral counselling that is worth considering. He states both are concerned with the care of others but the first is like that of a general practitioner and the latter is akin to that of a consultant.

There has been a scant number of studies that have addressed special aspects of the pastoral role in relation to this, for example: whilst providing counselling as a specific element of their ministry (Holaday et al., 2001); when working as chaplains (Taylor et al., 2006; Galek et al., 2011; Levy et al., 2011); when providing training for clergy on sexual misconduct (Pfeil, 2006); as part of a trauma team during a terrorist event (Gibson & Iwaniec, 2003). However, Hendron (2013) provided a wider understanding of the impact of working with human crisis within the daily pastoral ministry.

When it comes to clergy involvement in human crisis and trauma Weaver et al. (1996) argues that caring for those who have experienced psychological trauma is a significant part of the pastoral role. Whilst this book acknowledges many clerics may contest that they never have been nor potentially never will be involved in major trauma incidents, it is suggested that vicarious exposure does not necessarily need to be within major national or international disasters or trauma events. Nor indeed does the involvement need to take place within events that the majority may not immediately define as traumatic. Trauma is both personal and subjective to those who experience it. As such, events that some may see as merely difficult can in fact be life-changing for others.

It is recognised that frequently during critically distressing times clergy often remain an initial source of help that many individuals turn to even if at other points in their lives faith appears to be of less importance (Rudolfson & Tidefors, 2009). Mannon & Craword's (1996) work examined experiences by the clergy within the supportive element of their ministry and suggests for 42% of individuals with problems, a member of the clergy is the first port of call. Indeed Cole (2010) whilst attempting to conceptualise what makes care pastoral, suggests the tasks clergy undertake within their daily pastoral ministry are often difficult to distinguish from those of social workers, therapists, medical staff and counsellors. Evidence supporting this has emerged in incidents such as; the attacks in New York City on September 11th 2001 (Roberts et al., 2003; Flannelly et al., 2005); following natural disasters (Chinnici, 1985); working with sexual abuse victims (Rudolfsson & Tidefors, 2009); caring for survivors of human created atrocities such as war (Jacob, 1983); torture victims (Lernoux, 1980) and survivors of the death camps of World War II (Cohen, 1989).

That clergy are often sought out at times such as these should come as little surprise. Indeed Sigmund (2003) proposed the experience of trauma often causes an individual to seek, explore and question spiritual issues. This drive by many to bring religion and spirituality along side events happening in their lives has been aligned to an individual's need for a sense of coherence in their lives and their psychological wellbeing and this coherence appears to be dependent in some way on how we interpret events in our lives (Janoff-Bulmann, 1985). Adams (1995) argues that for many individuals their world-view, their methods of making meaning and extracting positivity from trauma are viewed as a spiritual process, even though this spirituality may not be tied to religion or even to conscious thought. In relation to traumatic, distressing or life altering events, one can begin to understand why individuals need to make some order out of chaos and it appears the aligning of these events within the framework of the will and power of a higher authority can allow individuals to formulate meaning and order from such events. Herman (1992) argues that when we fail to find meaning in trauma then this lack of meaning can result in the individual questioning the fundamental underpinnings of their belief systems. It has been identified that the holding of religious beliefs can assist in an individual being able to cope better with illness and has been associated with better health outcomes (Garter et al., 1991; Koenig et al., 2001). Considering these suggestions, it is hardly surprising to hear Everly's (2000) proposal that it is commonly observed in times of crisis, many individuals seek the help of religious and spiritual leaders. In fact, Francis & Lankshear, (1992) state:

> *"The top priority ascribed to the clergy is neither as spiritual director, religious educator nor community leader, but as a social carer. First and foremost churchgoers wish to see their clergy as exercising care over the aged, the lonely and the sick. The clergy are expected to combine the skills of social worker, health visitor and friendly neighbour."* (p19)

The Experiences of Ministry Project (COE, 2011) was a five-year longitudinal study undertaken by the Church of England. Whilst not specifically measuring the impact of trauma work, some of its findings in relation to the average hours' clergy reported exercising their pastoral duties (crisis and otherwise) are relevant for consideration. Full-time clergy reported spending an average of 5.1 hours per week; part-time 3.9; hospital chaplains 11.2 and dual post role 5.2 on pastoral duties. This study also highlights these means are on a par with other clergy duties such as preaching and liturgical duties and were only exceeded by those related to time undertaking administrative and organisational duties.

As previously stated, the thesis that provided the basis for this book explored the experiences of clergy within the island of Ireland. It was surprising to find a lack of empirical interest in relation to Irish clergy given Northern Ireland's bloody past and at times violent present and the fact that despite experiencing a process of peace spanning over 20 years, Northern Ireland remains characterised by a "*not-war-not peace*" situation (Sluka, 2009, p279). Additionally, it has been argued that this dichotomy of existence has not removed the suffering and traumatisation associated with the troubles, leading McAloney et al. (2009) to propose that both the psychological and social legacy of over thirty years of conflict has been passed on to post conflict generations, and the prevalence of violence remains at the forefront of many communities. Those studies that do exist whilst not necessarily focusing the vicarious impact of this work upon clerics are extremely important as they offer valuable insights into the involvement of ministers and priests within critical incidents within their pastoral role. Lount & Hargie (1997) undertook an examination of critical incidents in which Irish Catholic priests were involved within their pastoral ministry. These authors remarked, despite the large numbers involved in the priesthood and the interpersonal nature of their tasks, little empirical examination to characterise these tasks had been undertaken. They reported counselling and its associated skills form an important aspect of the ministerial role. Priests were involved in a myriad of issues that the authors defined as problem focused, crisis and support situations. Problem focused included drug and alcohol issues whilst crisis situations were identified as suicide and death. Support situations involved concerns such as depression. Within this study substantial problems emerged in relation to priests' perceptions of their training and preparation within Seminary College for this aspect of their ministry. This lack of preparation is a problematic finding when standing alone but becomes more worrying when placed in juxtaposition with Lount & Hargie's (1997) argument that it would be virtually impossible to effectively carry out this element of their pastoral role without adequate communication and counselling skills in which they appear not to receive sufficient training. This conversation is continued by Lount & Hargie (1998) discussing training needs for Catholic priests and during this investigation the authors identify that seminary training in various areas appears inadequate, with some of the areas mentioned including caring for the grieving and those encountering marriage difficulties.

In a later study investigating the counselling type work of Catholic priests in Northern Ireland, O'Kane & Millar (2001) highlight clergy as a vital source of help for individuals and communities. Their work strove to identify the extent to which Catholic priests engaged in work that involved a counselling element. Findings were in line with those of Lount & Hargie (1997) in that they highlighted priests were involved in work with a counselling focus across a diverse range of problems, reporting involvement in numerous problematic issues, many of which were described as serious and complex. The issues of addiction, marital issues and bereavement were seen most frequently.

In relation to priests' training for this element for their work, the findings also concurred with those of Lount & Hargie (1997) in that priests reported dissatisfaction with training and preparation for this work leading these authors to contend that the hierarchy of the church needed to address this issue within their seminary training. However, it was interesting to note that despite substantial issues around their training for this element of their ministry, many of the respondents expressed confidence in what they did. This finding appeared to reflect that of Mannon & Crawford (1996) who suggested that confidence displayed by clergy may be false and founded more on their unawareness of their limitations and less upon their actual abilities, leading O'Kane & Millar to assert that the inequitable picture between training and confidence urgently required further exploration.

Following on, O'Kane & Millar (2002) focused upon the methods and skills Catholic priests employ when responding to those who seek their help. Results indicated priests' involvement in problem solving across a wide range of issues. Priests' responses to these situations spanned the chasm between offering simple suggestions to taking on the task of solving problems. The number one problem-solving situation identified involved priests' perceptions that they were expected to solve the problem. It is hardly surprising that O'Kane & Millar (2002) contend that this perception places immense pressure upon the cleric to produce a solution.

Priests also indicated that listening to the experiences of others formed a large part of this work. This suggests that for some priests, the act of listening may have involved exposure to distressing accounts and details. Once again, the lack of training and support structures to assist priests in this work were evident and yet despite this, priests appeared not to have taken any independent steps to address the deficit. In the main the study highlights questions regarding priests' ability to carry out this work effectively.

In a wider context, accessing clergy during times of international and national crisis has been documented and is particularly evident during more recent world events such as those unfolding in New York on Sept 11th, 2001. Schuster at al. (2001) commented that in response to the events of September 11th in New York, 90% of Americans turned to religion as a coping response. Bradfield et al. (1989) in their study examining the role of clergy in response to the 1985 floods in West Virginia, reported in rural areas, where mental health resources are scarce, the clergy serve a "*particularly vital function in helping those who have had traumatic experiences*" (p397). The findings of this study highlighted that whilst clergy are not counsellors or mental health therapists, they may be accessed in these capacities by those they care for, especially when other professional resources are not within easy access.

Evidence points towards clergy being accessed not only during major international and national events but also in relation to more social and personal issues. Mental and emotional problems have been identified as one domain where their help is sought and they have been shown to play an important role in the management of these issues. Matthews (2007), examining the treatment models of Singapore clergy for mental health issues, commented clergy are recognised by those within their faith communities as important sources in the care of mental health. In a discussion paper expounding the potential benefits of including social workers as part of a pastoral team within the Catholic church Ebear et al. (2008) advocate Catholic priests have always done more than meet purely spiritual needs within their parishes and therefore the addition of a social worker as part of the pastoral team could further enhance the work undertaken. Weaver et al. (1996) found clergy have also been reported to respond to a wide range of incidents, which may include stressors that can precipitate PTSD, (Post-Traumatic Stress Disorder).

Leavey et al. (2007) examined clergy contact with those who experience mental illness. This was a valuable study as it explored not only Christian faith leaders, but also those from other faith backgrounds. These authors reported clergy play a valuable role in relation to this work and yet the significance of their contribution is not always recognised by those responsible for their training and care. Clergy reported they often feel fearful and lack confidence in these encounters, which is hardly surprising given they are potentially not adequately prepared for them and indicated at times they perceived their involvement in this work was detrimental to their key role as spiritual leaders. This led to challenges in integrating the religious and secular elements of their ministry.

The role of clergy within specific personal and social issues has also been highlighted. Examining acts of confiding in the clergy by those experiencing intimate partner violence, Neergaard et al. (2007) reported clergy are frequently accessed for this issue and females who are involved in intimate partner violence frequently attend religious services. Their data also indicated women attending these services were more likely to perceive clergy as being valuable and are therefore more likely to confide in them. These authors advocate for some clerics intimate partner violence may be the most challenging mental health problem they will face. Additionally, the counselling offered by clergy in these instances might have a positive influence on the psychological outcomes of the females involved in destructive relationships. These findings have important implications in that they not only highlight the involvement of the clergy within this sensitive and traumatic experience, but they also highlight the positive impact of their involvement.

Rudolfsson & Tidefors (2009) examined clergy readiness to meet the needs of victims of sexual abuse amongst a sample of Swedish clergy. Their findings reported those belonging to Christian congregations often access their cleric as a first means of support. 77% of respondents had experience of either disclosure of sexual abuse or caring for those who had undergone abuse. This level of involvement is worrying when coupled with the result that 24% of respondents did not feel confident in finding support within their church when undertaking this work. The authors identified adequate preparation for such work as a salient requirement of clergy training.

In light of the findings highlighting clergy are involved in a range of crisis issues, it is valuable to examine the cooperation between clergy and other helping agencies. Oppenheimer et al. (2004) undertook a search of the psychological literature to gain knowledge regarding the working association between clergy and psychologists. This search highlighted several valuable points and underpinned the findings of an earlier study several of the authors had undertaken (Weaver et al., 2003). Six major themes were identified within secular and religious journals during the period 1970-1999. These were: clergy are frontline workers with trauma; the need for more education; obstacles to collaboration; salience of shared values; benefits of collaboration and the role of clergy in prevention of crisis issues. Their search revealed clergy are more likely than mental health therapists to be asked for help from severely mentally distressed individuals (Hohmann & Larson, 1993). This was not surprising given clergies identified accessibility (Weaver et al., 2002) and the high degree of trust Americans have in them (Gallup & Lindsay, 1999).

The issue of lack of training, both on the part of clergy and psychologists was examined. Leading the authors to propose clergy appear to receive little or no training for undertaking this work. Whilst on the other hand psychologists had little understanding of spiritual issues. This lack of understanding was perhaps reflected in the process of referrals, which were identified as being mainly one directional, going from clergy to psychologists, with psychologists appearing more reticent to refer their clients on to clergy. This, the authors suggested, reflected psychologists being less willing to accept their clients as having problems which require a dimension of spiritual assistance. Additionally, the issue of differing values was raised, with clergy expressing the concern their faith and beliefs were being undermined by mental health professionals (Mannon & Crawford, 1996).

Oppenheimer et al.'s (2004) study is valuable not only as a resource for examining collaboration between clergy and mental health professionals, but as an indicator of the key role clergy play within their communities in relation to being accessed during times of crisis. Their findings added support to Weaver's (1995) call that mental health professionals need to recognise the role that the clergy play in both the screening and the follow-up care of trauma survivors. In their 2001 Suicide Prevention Strategy, the United States Department of Health went some way in acknowledging this when they identified clergy as often being 'gatekeepers' for those who suffer from mental health issues.

This chapter set out to explore the work of the pastoral ministry, especially in relation to studies examining clergy involvement with crisis issues. It has highlighted that clergy are involved within crisis work and that research appears to be taking an interest in the act of undertaking this work, but perhaps not necessarily focusing on its impact. One can surmise the increase in research interest in this area may be due in part to what Sigmund (2003) identifies as an increasing awareness of the importance of spirituality in the process of understanding and dealing with trauma. It has been documented that religious belief and behaviours can assist individuals to cope better and can also lead to enhanced health outcomes (Koenig

1992; Koenig et al., 2001). Therefore, those who use spirituality as a coping strategy may be more inclined to access faith leaders about their crisis issues. Specifically, in relation to the work of Irish clergy, the review indicated several valuable studies have emerged in relation to Catholic priests. More specifically it has highlighted specific aspects of the pastoral ministry which appear to firmly place clerics in the role of providing care and support for individuals and communities as they face life's challenges. Given that we now understand clergy are at risk then the following chapters will examine the basic concepts of that risk and what is known more generally about clergy psychological wellbeing.

Chapter 3

Understanding the Concepts: Vicarious Trauma, Secondary Traumatic Stress, Compassion Fatigue & Burnout

Smith (2004) proposes that the first step in the discussion of any construct is to provide a wider framework to place the construct in for discussion. Often in an attempt to understand a concept we are required to look backwards and seek out where its origins lie and secondary traumatic impact is no different. As such this chapter will take that required 'step back' and firstly discuss the wider concept of trauma as this will provide a sound foundation for understanding the subsequent related concept of secondary impact from trauma work. The chapter then moves on to provide a detailed exploration of the concepts associated with vicarious exposure to trauma: Vicarious Traumatisation and Secondary Traumatic Stress, also known as Compassion Fatigue. Finally, it briefly discusses the associated concept of Burnout as that has previously been of interest of clergy populations. A comprehensive account of the aetiology of each concept as presented within the literature together with the accompanying symptomatology is set out. The chapter also draws attention to the prevalence of this type of impact amongst a diverse range of professions. These professions are included as many of them undertake work that officially or unofficially may at times fall under the remit of the pastoral ministry and therefore merit examination within this book.

It is a tragic but unavoidable fact of life that trauma occurs. For some the experience is felt through illness, accident or through the death of a loved one. For others, the experience may come through the forces of nature or at the hands of other individuals. Herman (1992) attempts to distinguish between natural and human disasters,

> *"At the moment of trauma, the victim is rendered helpless by the overwhelming force. When the force is that of nature, we speak of disaster. When the force is that of other human beings, we speak of atrocities"* (p38).

Anna Freud (1969) argues that the term trauma is overused and should be reserved for events that are, "*shattering, devastating, causing internal disruption by putting ego functioning and ego mediation out of action*" (p242). Such statements merely highlight the difficulties encountered when defining such emotionally subjective matter. The term trauma originated in the Greek word '*traumat*', meaning wound and has several definitions.

"An injury (as a wound) to living tissue caused by an extrinsic agent; a disordered psychic or behavioural state resulting from severe mental or emotional stress or physical injury; an emotional upset; the personal trauma of an executive who is not living up to his own expectations" (Merriam-Webster, 2009).

When defining trauma, it is often described in terms of the traumatic events that cause it, yet Yule (2000) argues that by using the term *'traumatic event'* the extent of the trauma experienced is attributed to the event itself rather than the trauma being defined in its own terms (p10). Yule further argues that this presents a rather outdated understanding of the psychological distress that emerges. Van der Kolk (1987) offers some clarification on the subject stating:

"Trauma occurs when one loses the sense of having a safe place to retreat within or outside of oneself to deal with frightening emotions or experiences. This results in a state of helplessness, a feeling that one's actions have no bearing on the outcome of one's life" (p.31).

This proposal shifts the core of the trauma away from the actual event and places it within the individual's interpretation and personal significance. This insight is imperative given that the individual's interpretation of the event may indeed differ somewhat from the event itself and the individual's perception of the event will be coloured by such factors as the personal significance, consequences and implications arising from the situation.

The American Psychological Association's Diagnostic and Statistical Manual of Mental Disorders (DSM-IV-TR) definition of trauma is often used. It defines trauma as:

i.   *Persons experiencing, witnessing or confronting an event or events which involved actual or threatened death or serious injury, or a threat to the physical integrity of self or others.*

ii. *A person's response, which involves intense fear, helplessness or horror.*

iii. *Learning about unexpected or violent death, serious harm, or threat of death or injury by a family member or other close associate. (American Psychiatric Association, 2000).*

The American Psychiatric Association took a major step in recognising that one may be traumatised either directly or indirectly by vicariously witnessing another's trauma with the DSM-III-R (APA, 1987) expanding the criteria of trauma to include those events that are learned about by someone else who does not necessarily witness the direct event.

However, Levine (2005) advocates that not all trauma must result from a major catastrophe but may emerge from seemingly minor events and suggests a traumatic reaction depends as much on the individual's perception of the event as the event itself and therefore what may appear less significant for one individual may be catastrophic for another. This argument sits well with the ethos of this book wherein the experience of trauma and secondary trauma are presented as subjective and not translated in the same way by everyone.

The field of traumatology experienced an emergence of new interest in the mid-1980's, with the following decades witnessing the birth of several conceptualisations attempting to capture the experiences of those working with or caring for traumatised individuals and communities. Recognition of the existence of occupational stress syndromes had emerged in previous decades with discussions and gathering evidence regarding the stress and burnout syndromes and it was proposed these workers could experience depletion in their emotional and motivational resources resulting for some in exit from their roles (Freudenberger, 1974; Maslach, 1978). It is hardly surprising then that earliest interest in the difficulties which individuals experience within the course of their trauma work arose from anecdotal evidence from the workplace (Maslach et al., 2001). The cumulative effect of this has led to a growing acceptance of such experiences and it is now recognised that there is an inherent risk of emotional, cognitive and behavioural changes in the professional through indirect exposure to client's trauma (McBride, 2007). Furthermore, this impact can take its toll not only on individuals but also on their organisations.

In relation to secondary impact, calls emerged for recognition that those providing care for individuals who had experienced trauma could absorb some of the pain and suffering felt by those they care for (Figley, 1989,1993, 1995, 1996, 2002a; McCann & Pearlman, 1990a; Pearlman & Saakvitne, 1995a). The result of this recognition is a growing body of research which explores and attempts to capture the experiences of those involved in this caring and emotionally challenging work. It is now widely accepted that the impact of a client's narrative re-enactment of their traumatic experience can profoundly affect their therapist (Harrison & Westwood, 2009). Devilly et al. (2009) propose it makes intuitive sense to accept that there will be an impact on an individual's emotional experience either on a conscious or subconscious level when one is engaged in an empathic relationship which involves the identification and understanding of defensive reactions to other's emotional experiences.

Vulnerability to this transfer of trauma occurs in occupations that expose their practitioners to victimised and traumatised individuals and communities (Shah et al., 2007) or when working in situations where empathic engagement is of paramount importance to both the therapeutic relationship and the outcome (Sexton, 1999; Hunter & Schofield, 2006). Rothschild & Rand (2006) suggest there are two risk categories for secondary trauma, those who are close family members or associates of those who experience primary trauma and those who provide professional care and support for these individuals.

Earliest interest in the difficulties which individuals experience within the course of their trauma work arose from anecdotal evidence from the workplace (Maslach et al., 2001). This has led to a growing acceptance of these experiences and it is now recognised that there is an inherent risk of emotional, cognitive and behavioural changes in the professional through indirect exposure to client's trauma (McBride, 2007). Furthermore, this impact can take its toll not only on individuals but also on their organisations, resulting in decreased productivity, increased absenteeism and high staff turnover (Pfifferling & Gilley, 2000). However, the road to reaching this point of understanding has not been an easy one as not all agree such experiences exist and challenges to their existence have been raised. Dunkley & Whelan (2006) argue the development of knowledge has been hampered by a shortage of empirical research combined with a focus upon a limited range of professions and uncertainty regarding the factors associated with the experience.

Studies such as Sabin-Farrell & Turpin's (2003) examined the implications of secondary trauma upon the mental health of mental health workers and concluded that evidence supporting the existence of vicarious trauma was both meagre and inconstant. This did little to quench the flames of indecision and disagreement and led Sprang et al., (2007) to propose that, several decades after the emergence of the topic of secondary impact, contentions prevail around conceptual clarity. In trying to redirect attention away from confirming the existence of the experience and towards providing agreement on terminology Stamm (1999) advocated that less emphasis should be placed upon acceptance that this experience exists but instead the focus should be placed upon what it should be called. The formulation of this chapter revealed there still appears to have been little advance in resolving this issue.

Transference of the effects of trauma from one individual to another has been compared to the infectious nature of disease (Arvay, 2001). Mollica (1988) warns that those who care for traumatised individuals are at risk of becoming infected. The adverse consequences resulting from working with those who have experienced trauma have been assigned a range of conceptual labels:

- Vicarious traumatisation (McCann & Pearlman, 1990a)

- Secondary traumatic stress/compassion fatigue (Figley, 1993,1995)

- Burnout (Freudenberger, 1974; Maslach, 1976)

In an attempt to capture the positive consequences of trauma work Stamm (2002) added to the debate with the introduction of Compassion Satisfaction, suggesting that there can be a positive aspect to undertaking trauma work.

These diagnostic labels appear at times to overlap within their aetiology and symptomatology leading Sexton (1999) to propose that the terms are often used interchangeably without distinguishing what they are clearly describing. There is a consensus that empirical research on the definitive factors contributing to the associated conditions remains sparse (Avary, 2001; Figley, 2002a, 2002b; Pearlman, 2003) leading Devilly et al. (2009) to contend that whilst many professionals appear to simply assume that such concepts exist, there has been scant empirical evidence to support these assumptions. Baird & Kracen's (2006) synthesis of the concepts of vicarious trauma and secondary traumatic stress concluded that due to the lack of empirical research examining the differences between these concepts a lack of conceptual clarity remains. Motta (2008) contributes to this conversation noting that whist the concept of secondary impact is now accepted there remains a scarcity of well-grounded empirical evidence.

Figley (2002a) contends that recognition by the American Psychiatric Association that an individual could become impacted by another's traumatic material has, rather than providing clarity, added to the confusion. He suggests the inclusion of secondary impact has resulted in a '*conceptual conundrum*' (p4) within the field. This lack of clarity he argues has resulted from the existence of several concepts, which appear to represent different yet associated phenomenon and which he contends few studies have identified or separated. Studies of prevalence levels have provided insights into the impact of working with trauma and crisis across diverse populations. However, there appear to be problematic issues in relation to this body of knowledge as at times particular studies state they are examining one concept whilst describing the theoretical framework of another, leaving the readers confused as to which aspect of the experience is being discussed or measured and an expanding range of instruments to capture measurement of impact has further compounded the situation. Sabin-Farrell & Turpin (2003) highlighted this state of affairs proposing the inter-changeable use of terms has made discrimination between concepts difficult within the literature.

Some attempts have been made to offer clarity between the concepts. Jenkins & Baird (2002) clearly state that despite conceptual similarities in impact upon the professional, the emphasis of Vicarious Traumatisation, Secondary Traumatic Stress and Burnout clearly differ. Vicarious Traumatisation relates to distortions in cognitive schemas whilst Secondary Traumatic Stress shares similar symptomatology to Post Traumatic Stress Disorder (PTSD), with both focusing on trauma exposure. Burnout on the other hand conceptualises a negative response to pressures within the organisational environment but these do not focus specifically on trauma. Bride et al. (2007) discussing the subject suggest that despite differences between the terms Secondary Traumatic Stress and Vicarious Traumatisation in theoretical origin and symptom foci, they are both terms that describe the negative impact experienced by professionals through working with traumatised clients.

Van der Kolk & McFarland (1996) observe that, "*In important ways, an experience does not really exist until it can be named and placed into larger categories*" (p4). This statement resonated with the author in that for many who assist those who are traumatised, the experiences they subsequently endure may involve more than one element identified within existing literature. Therefore, for the purpose of this book the range of terms employed within the literature are examined and the following definitions are accepted as strands of these experiences.

- Secondary traumatic stress/compassion fatigue is presented as a set of symptoms which are almost identical to those of PTSD although lesser in their intensity and include intrusion, hyper-arousal and avoidance (Figley, 1995,1996, 2002a).

- Vicarious traumatisation is used to define increasing distortions upon the professional cognitive schemas in relation to themselves, others and the world (McCann & Pearlman, 1990b).

- Compassion satisfaction embraces the positive feelings emerging when working with those in need (Stamm, 2002, 2009).

- Burnout is used to capture the feelings of emotional exhaustion, depersonalisation and reduced personal accomplishment associated with one's work environment (Maslach, 1976).

Attempts to conceptualise the phenomena of secondary impact amongst the helping professions emerged in the early 1990's. McCann & Pearlman (1990a) were some of the first to identify this impact presenting their term Vicarious Traumatisation as representing the negative experiences of therapists who worked with traumatised clients. Their initial work emerged from their own professional experiences and focused upon those working with adult survivors of sexual abuse and presented Vicarious Traumatisation as an experience that was interactive, cumulative, negative and inevitable for those working within this profession (McCann & Pearlman, 1990b, 1990c). Earlier literature around the topic referred to this impact as being either a type of burnout or a counter-transference reaction, however Vicarious Traumatisation is presented as being specific to the client's presentation of traumatic material and specific to those involved in listening to it (McCann & Pearlman, 1990a, 1990b).

McCann & Saakvitne (1995) postulated therapists working with survivors of trauma experience pervasive and enduring changes to their cognitive schemas, which in turn impact upon their feelings, relationships and wider existence. The extent to which these changes can be destructive to both the therapist and the therapeutic process will depend upon the individual therapist's ability to engage in a process of integration and transformation of their client's traumatic events. Pearlman & Mac Ian (1995) propose that by listening to a client's explicit and disturbing material, the therapist becomes a witness to their traumatic event. The experience of impact is presented as so intense that it involves; "*profound changes in the core aspects of the therapist's self*" (Pearlman & Saakvitne, 1995a, p152) and these changes cause disruptions in the professional's cognitive schemas of identity, memory and belief systems. Therefore, Vicarious Traumatisation represents the professional's reactions to their client's raw traumatic material over a sustained period and encompasses the individual's subsequent cognitive disruptions. It is this repeated exposure that can cause a shift in the way an individual perceives themselves, others and the world around them (Trippany et al., 2004).

Emergence of this concept has proved a complex approach to the understanding of professionals' reactions to their client's trauma (Trippany et al., 2004). Two of the earliest studies in this area (Pearlman & Mac Ian, 1995; Schauben & Frazier, 1995) are often cited as the main source of evidence for the development of the concept amongst professionals who work with traumatised individuals (Vrklevski

& Franklin, 2008). These early studies identified that therapists with less professional experience reported higher disruptions in beliefs associated with trust, safety, control, intimacy and self-esteem. They also cited differences between therapists who had a personal history of trauma and those who had not. However there remains a lack of consensus as other studies have failed to replicate this association (Lerias & Byrne, 2003).

McCann & Pearlman, (1990a, 1990b, 1990c) contend the theoretical basis for Vicarious Traumatisation lies within Constructivist Self-Development Theory and this theory offers valuable insights. Constructivist Self-Development Theory carries an underlying assumption that reaction to and adaption of an individual's experience of trauma lies within a complex interwoven tapestry encompassing the individual's personality, personal history, the traumatic event itself and the cultural and social context in which the event takes place. Its underlying assumptions are based on earlier constructivist work, which suggested that individuals construct and construe their own realities (Epstein, 1985; Piaget, 1971). Janoff-Bulman (1985) identified three basic beliefs that are impacted and altered by trauma: the belief that oneself is invulnerable; the belief that the world is just and meaningful and a positive view of oneself. The theory contends that individual differences in adaptation exist and as such argues that as information and experience of an event are incorporated into an individual's belief and meaning system, they result in a representation of the survivor's experience rather than an objective forensic representation of the trauma event.

Constructivist Self-Development Theory offers a basis for understanding the psychological, interpersonal and transpersonal impact of traumatic life events upon an individual and is a framework wherein one can grasp a better understanding of the impact of trauma upon the helping professional. Furthermore, it emphasises the adaptive function of individual beliefs in addition to the individual's style of affect management (Pearlman & Saakvitne, 1990a, 1990b).

Constructivist Self-Development Theory has been presented to explain the changes occurring in both the individual's cognitive schemas and their perceptions of reality, which occur due to the interactions of the client's material and the professional's personal characteristics (Saakvitne & Pearlman, 1996). It is this self-development process in which individuals remain active in the creation of their own perceptions of reality and is viewed as a style of adaptive affect management. Therefore, intuitively one can begin to understand how being exposed to the experience of other's traumatic events can result in the production of another unique representation of what has taken place.

Pearlman & Saakvitne (1995b) identify five components of the self within Constructivist Self-Development Theory. These are presented below

Frame of Reference	This involves a meaningful frame of reference and is proposed by McCann & Pearlman (1990b) to represent a fundamental human need. This is normally defined as the framework wherein an individual's understanding of the world is constructed (Pearlman & Saakvitne, 1995b). Beneath its umbrella lies an individual's worldview and belief system and therefore it is a fundamental part of the process of understanding one's self and the wider world. If this frame of reference is disturbed in any way then the consequences can seep into the helping relationship. For example, a counsellor with a distorted frame of reference, dealing with a victim of rape, may find they believe the victim was to blame.
Self-Capacities	This encompasses capabilities that allow the individual to preserve a reliable rational sense of self-identity, connection and positive self-esteem (Pearlman & Saakvitne, 1995b). These self-capacities allow the individual to manage emotions and sustain positive feelings regarding themselves and consequently to successfully manage relationships with others. When these self-capacities are disrupted the individual may experience a loss of their own identity, they may experience interpersonal difficulties and find themselves increasingly unable to manage, or even be exposed to, negative emotions. This disruption can result in the individual feeling unable to meet the needs of others and may manifest itself in the individual actively avoiding any exposure to negative emotions.
Ego Resources	These permit the individual to meet their psychological needs and enables them to relate interpersonally with others (Pearlman & Saakvitne, 1995b). Aspects of these abilities have been identified as being able to conceive consequences, to set boundaries and to self-protect. If one's ego resources are disrupted, the results may be over perfectionism, loss of empathic ability and over extension within the work environment.
Psychological Needs & Cognitive Schemas	The fourth and fifth components involve psychological needs and the cognitive schemas. Herein lies the needs of individuals in the areas of safety, trust, intimacy and control. These are all proposed as being basic human psychological needs in addition to being how individuals process information relating to these needs in the development of their cognitive schemas regarding themselves and others (Pearlman & Saakvitne, 1995b).

Pearlman & Saakvitne (1995b) present a number of factors associated with therapists' vulnerability to, or resilience against, Vicarious Traumatisation:

- Exposure to trauma patients

- Therapist's own personal history of trauma

- The individual's personal capacity for emotional empathy

- Spirituality

Examination of existing empirical studies on vicarious trauma has revealed several points of interest that appear to both confirm and contradict these proposals. Researchers have identified that the degree of exposure to traumatised clients may predispose a therapist to vicarious trauma (Brady et al., 1999; Chrestman, 1995; Pearlman & Mac Ian, 1995). Arvay's (2001) study suggested the number of traumatised clients in a therapist's case load, exclusively working with traumatised clients, years of clinical experience and the therapist's education level all appeared to be influential in the development of secondary impact. In a more recent study Vrkelevski & Franklin (2008) found than lawyers who dealt with criminal cases reported higher levels of Vicarious Traumatisation than solicitors who dealt with non-criminal cases. However, other studies have found no support for this association, for example Kadambi (2004) reported no difference in levels of vicarious impact between trauma and non-trauma therapists.

Pearlman & Saakvitne (1995a; 1995b) identify personal trauma history as a predisposing factor of Vicarious Traumatisation which suggests that encounters with the tragedies of others can cause personal traumatic memories that have not been fully assimilated into one's cognitive schemas to resurface. The literature has produced mixed findings for this factor. Some have found associations between personal experiences of trauma and levels of impact (Follette et al., 1994; Pearlman & Mac Ian, 1995), whilst others offer no such support (Schauben & Frazier, 1995).

Empathy is presented within the literature as a necessary yet potentially detrimental ability for the therapist and a landscape is painted where the more empathically engaged a therapist is with a client the more vulnerable they are to vicarious trauma (Pearlman & Saakvitne, 1995b, 1995c; Sexton, 1999). Rothschild & Rand (2006) provide valuable insight here by stating the understanding of another's pain is not the same as feeling this pain. Indeed, understanding pain is necessary in order to help but feeling pain can hinder and be detrimental to the helping process. The emergence of Harrison & Westwood's (2009) study yielded novel findings in relation to the associations between empathy and secondary traumatisation. Examining protective factors against vicarious impact their findings indicated that rather than being a risk factor, professionals identified a deep empathic engagement, defined by them as, "*exquisite empathy*" (p 207), as potentially a protective factor. Their findings appear to 'fly in the face' of existing studies and not only present exciting opportunities for future research but also pose some serious questions regarding the implications for practice.

Spirituality as a protective factor in health has been explored previously in literature. Morgan (2004) argues that, '*If a person's spiritual needs fail to be addressed, a person's emotional well-being is put at risk*' (p8). It is important to highlight that spirituality and religion, whilst sharing similarities are not the same concept. Smith & Orlinsky (2004) presents spirituality as having broader parameters than formal religion and this thought process is emulated by Pearlman

& Saakvitne, (1995a) who portray spirituality as a general term encompassing aspects such as hope, faith, joy, forgiveness, creativity and acceptance and potentially representing a belief in a higher power, which is not necessarily represented by a deity.

Associations between spirituality, wellbeing and coping have previously been explored. Cooper (2003) found that both spiritual and religious involvement are positively related to health and inversely related to maladaptive coping strategies such as substance abuse and mental disorders. Graham et al. (2001) investigated the relationship between religion, spirituality and coping with stress and reported a positive relationship between spiritual wellbeing and immunity against stress. Tischler et al. (2002) suggest the literature pertaining to spirituality presents individuals who have healthier, happier lives and are more satisfied and productive at work whilst Flier (1995) proposed that spirituality offers individuals a completely different way to experiencing their work environment.

Pearlman & Saakvitne (1995a) propose that individuals who possess a '*larger sense of meaning and connection*' (p161) are less likely to experience a vicarious impact. Although conversely, they also suggest that Vicarious Traumatisation can result in a disruption of the individual's spirituality resulting in loss of hope, confusion, bewilderment and powerlessness. Pearlman & Mac Ian's (1995) study amongst trauma counsellors reported that 44% of their participants indicated their spirituality imparted them with an effective coping strategy when dealing with the potentially negative aspects of their work. These assertions supported the work of Wittine (1995) who reported counsellors possessing a stronger sense of spirituality were more likely to accept the realities of the human experience and accept their inability to personally alter these experiences.

Pearlman & Saakvitne (1995a, 1995b) propose Vicarious Traumatisation results in profound disruption in how an individual views, experiences and interprets the world. These disruptions alter the individual's frame of reference, identity, spirituality and worldview. This disruption to the sense of identity may result in the individual experiencing a feeling of un-realness to the world around them and may further lead to an affective numbness and distancing from others.

Disruptions in an individual's worldview alters their perception of how things happen, challenging belief systems and potentially leading the individual to feel sad and confused (Pearlman & Saakvitne, 1995a). Cranfield (2005) reviewing the literature concerning vicarious impact amongst therapists who treat traumatised patients contended that once affected, sufferers can begin to question the meaning and purpose of life. This loss of meaning is associated with the individual becoming cynical, believing nothing is worthwhile, feeling hopeless, outraged, experiencing emotional numbness and withdrawal (Herman, 1992; Pearlman & Saakvitne, 1995a).

In a later study Trippary et al. (2004) further supported the argument of spirituality as a protective factor by proposing that those at risk of impact can utilise whatever resource they find brings them a sense of meaning as a factor to help mediate the effects of the work they do. The summation of these studies would suggest clergy, through the very spiritual fabric of their role, might potentially be offered some immunity against the negative impact of trauma work.

The work of Chares Figley is seminal to understanding the impact of working with trauma. Much of his early work was undertaken with veterans of the Vietnam War (Figley, 1978). This involvement with veterans and their families led to his proposal that those who are exposed to such individuals, either through personal or professional encounters, are challenged through the work to confront their own vulnerability. In fact, Figley (1995) contends that the recorded number of victims impacted by traumatic events are gross underestimations as they only count the individual who was directly affected in the initial trauma and do not encompass all those who had been affected vicariously. Figley (1993, p7) introduced his concept of secondary traumatic stress as:

> *"The natural and consequent behaviours and emotions resulting from knowing about a traumatizing event experienced by a significant other the stress resulting from helping or wanting to help a traumatized or suffering person"*

Figley (1995) perceived this label presented a negative reflection on the individual's mental capacities and therefore was viewed as derogatory whilst the suggestion that one can experience fatigue or stress in the line of compassionate work sat more comfortably with descriptions of the causes and symptoms of this concept. Therefore, he subsequently introduced the term Compassion Fatigue as a more acceptable, interchangeable term for the condition. Figley (2002b) indicates:

> *"Compassion fatigue is a state of tension and preoccupation with the traumatized patients by re-experiencing the traumatic events, avoidance /numbing of reminders, persistent arousal associated with the patient. It is a function of being witness to the suffering of others"* (p1435)

Joinson (1992) previously coined the term 'compassion fatigue' during an investigation of burnout amongst nurses suggesting that the caring approach adopted by some nurses might lead to the absorption of the traumatic stress of those they help.

Figley's model is grounded within the symptomatology of Post-Traumatic Stress Disorder, wherein the individual may experience a range of biopsychosocial reactions including disturbing images, hyper-arousal, upsetting emotions, avoidance and an inability to function normally (Figley, 1995, 1996, 2002a, 2002b; Figley & Roop, 2006). The associations between the symptoms of Post-Traumatic Stress Disorder (APA, 2000) have been identified as almost identical to those of secondary impact although much less intense (Bride et al., 2007). Yet despite their similarity, Figley (1995) adamantly adheres to the philosophy that experiencing some level of impact from this work is a natural consequence and as such should not be presented as an abnormal or pathological reaction. This echoes Munroe's (1999) proposal that being impacted vicariously through another's trauma should be viewed as a natural occupational hazard. It is the individual's failure to address and manage signs of the experience, which may result in more detrimental long-term impact upon the individual (Radley & Figley, 2007).

Research findings have identified that specific fields of employment carry high risks for Secondary Traumatic Stress: child protection services (Dane, 2000); social workers (Adams et al., 2008); mental health workers (Meldrum et al., 2002); disaster response teams (Holtz et al., 2002); primary health care workers (Imai et al., 2004); oncology staff, (Sherman et al., 2006) and counsellors (Arvay, 2001).

Figley (1995,1996, 2002a) offers several explanations as to why some individuals are more deeply affected by their work with trauma sufferers than others and at the core of this are the concepts of exposure and empathy. He argues that if one is exposed to and involved in another's difficult experience then almost inevitability one will be affected on some level over the short or long term. Walker (2001) offers a beautiful conceptualisation of this through the suggestion that the painful secrets of a client may become the distressing secrets of a counsellor.

The relationship between levels of exposure to the traumatic material of others and the incidence of impact again generated inconclusive results. In their study Adams et al. (2008) examined the experiences of 236 social workers operating in the aftermath of the attacks of September 11th in New York. Their findings supported exposure to traumatised clients as a risk factor for compassion fatigue amongst social workers. Galek et al. (2011) examined Secondary Traumatic Stress amongst professional chaplains who provided counselling, reporting it to be positively associated with the number of hours spent counselling trauma victims. Laposa & Aldon (2005) examined the consequences of traumatic exposure amongst emergency nurses, with one group having direct (primary) exposure to a traumatic event and a second group having indirect (secondary) exposure. They reported no significant differences in levels of PTSD amongst the two groups as measured by the Post Traumatic Stress Diagnostic Scale (Foa et al., 1993).

However, Baird & Jenkins (2003) reported no association between levels of Secondary Traumatic Stress and the number of trauma clients or the hours per week worked with these individuals. Such mixed results led Phelps et al. (2009) to argue that not everyone who undertakes caring work is affected and therefore exposure alone is not a sufficient explanation as to why these conditions occur.

Figley (2002a) suggests the more inexperienced the individual is in working with trauma the more at risk they are. An inverse relationship between professional experience and trauma related symptoms has been reported. For example, Chrestman (1995) found correlations between higher levels of therapists' professional experience and decreased avoidance, anxiety and trauma symptoms. Although in relation to the previous risk factor of exposure, it could be argued that the more a therapist is exposed to trauma the more experience is gained and therefore one risk factor could potentially cancel out another. Additionally, it could be argued those who experienced especially high levels of impact may have already exited their role and are therefore not being accounted for within research.

Empathy is viewed as necessary for the therapeutic progress (Rogers, 1951), yet it sits in juxtaposition as a potential risk factor for the secondary impact (Figley, 1995). This presents those whose work requires 'empathic engagement' as a tool for approaching a problem from another's perspective with a 'catch 22' situation and it is here one begins to see the vulnerability of therapists, counsellors, medical staff and, as this book proposes, the clergy.

In an account of the demands, challenges and costs of the pastoral role Abernethy (2002) discusses vulnerability and empathy:

> *"Vulnerability is the ultimate mark of the ministry to those in crisis. To be vulnerable with them is part of our calling. To empathise with people and to try and discern their struggle is fundamental"* (p47).

Therefore, one can begin to understand how through the very nature of their calling, which demands them to 'come alongside' those who suffer, clergy are potentially at risk of negative impact. Surprisingly, empathy as a risk factor has been examined sparsely within the literature and the current review highlighted a distinct lack of research specifically examining empathy as a risk variable. Indeed, the concept of empathy is often paid lip service to within discussion articles and literature reviews yet there appears to be a lack of studies which have employed empathy specifically as a variable to correlate with secondary trauma scores. This was somewhat surprising in light of the core theorists' proposals that empathy puts professionals at risk of secondary impact (McCann & Pearlman, 1990b; Figley, 1995). Galek et al. (2011) echo this thought stating it is surprising that various degrees of empathy have not been examined in relation to secondary impact. In one of the few studies examining empathy Simon et al. (2005) reported that the emotionally intense interactions and the use of empathy between oncology social workers and their patients led to the increased secondary impact as measured in terms of Compassion Fatigue.

Figley (1995) proposes that individuals with personal experiences of trauma, especially if they have not succeeded in working through their experiences, could increase their susceptibility to negative impact. As we progress through life we encounter personally difficult and traumatic situations, which we may or may not deal with appropriately (Ramos et al., 2007). It is these unresolved issues he advocates which can resurface when listening to a client's traumatic material, resulting in the appearance of dramatic and sudden symptoms accompanied by little warning. Figley (2002a) suggests that life disruptions in terms of changes in personal or professional responsibility or life routine, whilst not responsible for the initial development of the experience, can when combined with other risk factors make the professional more vulnerable to its development.

Whilst many of the risk factors associated with Secondary Traumatic Stress are similar to those of Vicarious Traumatisation it is within its symptoms that differences emerge. Secondary Traumatic Stress does not specifically focus on the cognitive but encompasses a wider range of experiences, which mimic those associated with PTSD (Figley, 1995; Baird & Kracen, 2006). Figley (2002a) directed that primary and secondary traumatisation symptoms are similar and therefore their effects, such as hyper-arousal, exhaustion, avoidance and numbing, are difficult to distinguish, expect in intensity.

Secondary Traumatic Stress symptoms include re-experiencing the traumatic event, the occurrence of intrusive thoughts, avoidance or numbing behaviours in relation to reminders of the event, sleep disturbances, anxiety, loss of compassion and discouragement (Figley, 1995). The negative effects are also thought to impact the individual's ability to effectively assist those who seek their help (Figley, 1996, 1999; Najjar et al., 2009).

However, Figley (1995) suggests recovery normally involves a much shorter period of time than recovery from other conditions such as Vicarious Trauma and Burnout, suggesting that whilst they may be related phenomenon, they are distinct. Figley (1999) attempted to offer further clarification between a secondary traumatic stress reaction and a secondary traumatic stress disorder, stating symptoms with a duration of less than a month should be recognised as Secondary Traumatic Stress which is considered to be a normal crisis related reaction. However, if symptoms persist and extend beyond six months after the initial event that triggered them, they may be viewed as developing into secondary traumatic stress disorder. He further contends that this disorder is almost identical to Post Traumatic Stress Disorder, as defined within the DSM-IV-R (American Psychiatric Association, 2000) except that in the case of secondary traumatic stress disorder the trauma of the initial event is experienced second hand.

The growing body of knowledge related to the impact of working with trauma provides substantial evidence that there is indeed a cost to caring. Studies have examined levels of impact across a wide range of professional and non-professional groups. Baird & Kracen (2006) undertook a research synthesis of studies in the period 1994-2003 and reported investigations of Secondary Traumatic Stress amongst the following populations; sexual abuse counsellors (Follette et al., 1994; Simonds, 1996; Dickes, 1998; Brady et al., 1999; Young,1999; Trippary, 2000); clinical & counselling psychologists (Allt, 1999); trauma therapists (Pearlman & Mac Ian, 1995; Weaks, 1999; Myers & Cornelle, 2002); mental health professional (Price, 2001); mental health workers post September 11th attacks (Creamer, 2002); mental health workers following the Oklahoma City bombing (Wee & Myers, 2002) and professionals working with abused youth (Camerlengo, 2002).

Caring professional groups appear to be of interest to researchers and a number of studies have recently emerged within the nursing and related professions; heart and vascular nurses (Young et al., 2011); oncology nurses (Quinal et al., 2009); forensic nurses (Townsend & Campbell, 2009); midwives (Leinweber & Rowe, 2010) and hospice nurses & staff (Abendroth & Flannery, 2006; Robbins et al., 2009). Beck & Gable (2012) undertook a mixed methods study to determine the prevalence of Secondary Traumatic Stress amongst labour and delivery nurses and to explore their experiences during traumatic childbirth that delivered valuable insights into the challenges of this role. Employing the Secondary Traumatic Stress Scale (Bride et al., 2003) they revealed 355 of the nurses had high levels of Secondary Traumatic Stress. This quantitative element was further complemented by qualitative findings. Content analysis uncovered six major themes related to being present at traumatic births. The themes involved: factors that magnified exposure to traumatic births; struggles to remain professional during these experiences; agonising over how events should have been; being haunted by symptoms of Secondary Traumatic Stress and considerations of leaving their roles in order to survive.

Hardly surprisingly therapists and counsellors have come under the research lens. In one of the more recent studies, Craig & Sprang (2010) examined aspects of positive and negative impact amongst a sample of 532 trauma therapists. Employing the ProQOL III (Stamm, 2005) they found that only 5% of participants reported experiencing high level of Secondary Traumatic Stress above the cut off point indicated by Stamm. These authors also reported that utilising evidence based practice in the form of empirically tested interventions such as Cognitive Behavioural Therapy (CBT) to manage signs of the impact was a predictor for reducing secondary impact. Previously Arvay & Uhelmann (1996) examined a sample of 161 trauma counsellors in British Columbia and found 14% of their sample reported traumatic stress levels similar to PTSD. They also found 24% of the counsellors reported they felt life was stressful. These authors took the steps of offering a detailed 'profile' of what a traumatised counsellor looks like. This took the form of an individual in their early 40's, working in an agency with less than 10 years experience. They suggested this individual would have a high caseload (10-26 trauma clients) and their education would be less than Masters level.

Those who work with survivors of abuse have also proved a popular source of exploration (Chrestman, 1995; Kassan-Adams, 1995; Steed & Dowling, 1998; Brady et al., 1999; Ghahramanlou & Brodleck, 2000; Iliffe & Steed, 2000). This may be in part due to the concept of secondary impact emerging initially from the experiences of therapists working with survivors of sexual abuse. These studies primarily have employed a quantitative approach using varied instruments to measure symptomatic distress but their findings have come under criticism as being difficult to interpret with concerns also expressed over their sample size, instruments used and participant recruitment (Sabin-Farrell & Turpin, 2003).

Impact amongst social workers has also been explored with Bride et al. (2007) reporting that social workers are likely to be exposed to secondary trauma events through their work with clients. The same study indicated that a significant minority of the social workers involved in the sample, (approx 15%), were likely to meet the diagnostic criteria for PTSD. These findings offered support for the research by Siebert (2004) indicating that approx 19% of social workers in North Carolina, USA, meet the study criteria for depression.

Impact has also been explored among more diverse professions; solicitors (Vrklevski & Franklin, 2008); teachers (Lucas, 2008); judges (Jaffe et al., 2006) oncology nurses (Sinclair & Hamill, 2007) and telephone counsellors (Dunkley & Whelan, 2006). Other areas of interest have compared the impact between groups such as nurses and counsellors (Lyon, 1993), professionals and volunteers working with survivors of sexual victimisation (Salston & Figley, 2003), mental health professionals and police officers (Follette at al., 1994).

In the main studies have involved samples that are dominated by females: Jenkins & Baird (2002) used a sample of sexual and domestic violence counsellors, 95 female, 4 male; Slattery & Goodman (2009), Domestic violence advocates,

100% female; Buchanan et al. (2006), Canadian mental health workers, 84% female, 16% male; (Dunkley & Wheelan (2006), telephone counsellors, 88.7% female, 11.3% male and Vrklevski & Franklin (2008), solicitors, 64% female, 36% male. This skewed representation may be due to many of these professions being dominated by females. Furthermore, the review also indicated that qualitative explorations have been less prevalent and have not always involved face-to-face interviewing or focus groups.

Iliffe & Steed (2000) carried out semi-structured interviews with domestic violence counsellors, whilst in an earlier study Crothers (1995) interviewed those who worked with survivors of childhood trauma. However, other studies have had a qualitative element to them but did not necessarily employ interviews (Harrison & Westwood, 2009; Ortlepp & Friedman, 2002) instead often employing open-ended questions as part of their quantitative data collection. Often the qualitative element to these studies has informed more nuanced discussion of secondary impact, revealing issues which are pertinent, specific and personally salient for those who undertake this work.

The issue of Burnout has often been associated with the clergy role and as such it merits a brief inclusion within this chapter. The rationale behind this is that Burnout is at times viewed as the reason that clerics exit the ministry. However, there has been scant consideration of the vicarious impact of trauma work within this wider context. Interestingly, McCann & Pearlman (1990c) propose that the symptoms of Burnout may be the final result of continual exposure to traumatic events that one cannot assimilate or work through. Additionally, Figley (1995) contended that many people simply view the stresses associated with their role as Burnout. These statements suggest that Burnout may be the final destination in a journey in which secondary traumatisation may be a significant sojourner but a sojourner that potentially is not always recognised or considered (Hendron et al., 2012).

Burnout is conceptualised as a syndrome, which is the result of chronic interpersonal stressors involved in one's job (Maslach et al., 2001). Pines & Aronson (1988, p9) defined it as '*a state of physical, emotional and mental exhaustion caused by long term involvement in an emotionally demanding situation*'. Several conceptual differences exist between Burnout and the other conditions discussed in this chapter. Firstly, Burnout is viewed as a process rather than a specific fixed condition, which begins insidiously, progresses slowly and is cumulative (Maslach & Jackson, 1982; Cherniss, 1995) whereas a secondary trauma impact can be sudden and result from only one encounter (Figley, 1995). Secondly, Burnout is associated with stressors within one's job whilst secondary impact is a direct result of exposure to another's emotionally distressing material (Cranfield, 2005).

However, it is worth noting that the concept of Burnout did emerge from within the caring domains. Freudenberger (1974), a psychiatrist working within an alternative health care agency and Maslach (1976), a social psychologist whose interest lay in the arena of the emotions within the workplace conducted the early work on the concept. Freudenberger (1975) contributed direct personal accounts of his experiences and the experience of those who worked alongside him in relation to diminishing levels of motivation, commitment and emotion for their work.

Additionally, Maslach (1976) offered an expansive range of qualitative data derived from interviews with human service workers regarding the emotional challenges of their jobs. From these initial works it quickly became evident that the concept of Burnout had its roots within those occupations that involved a central core of providing care for others. It is the negative interpersonal aspect of these contributions which has set the tone for much of the subsequent work and has resulted in an array of diagnostic labels associated with the negative psychological effects experienced by the professional involved. Maslach et al., (2001) contend the connecting thread between these labels is that they are all viewed in terms of the individual's relational interactions in the workplace rather than their stress responses.

The concept of Burnout is now widely accepted as consisting of three components: emotional exhaustion, depersonalisation and reduced personal accomplishment/inefficacy. It is firmly identified as being related to the work situation in association with high levels of work stress and low rewards (Byre, 1994; Lee & Ashford, 1996; Maslach et al., 2001; Cranfield, 2005; Devilly et al., 2009). The individual involved may feel they have no control over their conditions within the work environment and that there exists no opportunity to achieve their work-related goals (Maslach et al., 2001). Whilst depression has been related to Burnout (Maslach et al., 1996), the work of Bakker et al. (2000) established that Burnout is specific to the work setting, whilst depression can encompass all aspects of an individual's life. The three components of burnout shall now be individually addressed:

The first, emotional exhaustion, was identified by Maslach & Jackson (1982) as the most outwardly visible warning sigh of the three components. The centrality of this component in the diagnosis of the condition has resulted in the argument by some that the other two components are virtually redundant (Shirom, 1989). This overwhelming feeling of exhaustion may be experienced as a depletion of an individual's emotional and physical resources whilst the individual's inability to muster any more emotional or physical resources is argued to represent the stress element of Burnout (Maslach et al., 2001).

Rella et al. (2009) investigated the progression of chronic maladaptive fatigue amongst nursing students when undertaking a three-year nursing degree course. Their findings showed the levels of maladaptive fatigue increased significantly as the course progressed, with 20% of final year students reporting serious signs of fatigue. These findings, whilst insightful, must be viewed with some caution as the study was not a longitudinal one but involved a sample taken from across the three years of the course and therefore the progression of fatigue was not plotted along personal three-year experiences.

Shirom (1989) and Maslach et al. (2001) both argue that to look at only the emotional exhaustion aspect, especially out of context, could lead one to totally lose sight of the entire concept of Burnout as it only represents one aspect of stress and does not address the complexity of relationships that individuals may have with their jobs.

The second component is depersonalisation wherein an individual may have feelings of cynicism and detachment from their job and the individuals they are required to interact with, representing the interpersonal element of the construct. It is here that one may become callous or even totally removed from certain aspects of one's role or treat those with whom they interact as impersonal objects (Maslach et al., 2001).

Freudenberger (1990) suggested those who enter the caring profession with enthusiasm and real vitality for their work often become cynical and depressed. They can experience feelings of helplessness and frustration at times and this may be exhibited as anger. This anger may be directed towards the work environment in general or the client in particular. If not recognised and successfully addressed, these feelings can result in the professional becoming either physically or mentally unable to carry out their work. Doolittle (2007) examined Burnout and coping amongst parish-based clergy and reported higher spirituality was positively correlated to higher depersonalisation. He proposed either an individual's relationship with God may lead to a more objectified view of mankind or alternatively, due to their spiritual based centre, an individual may be less attached to the world.

Finally, the third element is reduced personal accomplishment/inefficacy where there may exist a sense of ineffectiveness and lack of achievement of goals around an individual's work role. This final symptom represents the self-evaluation element of Burnout as one experiences feelings of inadequacy, incompetence and a failed sense of achievement in the course of their work. It has been argued that this element is reflective of the combination of cynicism and exhaustion (Byrne, 1994; Lee & Ashford, 1996).

There is increasing evidence that Burnout is multidimensional in nature and the factors that contribute to its progression stem from the intrapersonal, interpersonal and organisational spheres (Truchot et el., 2000). For example, higher levels of education are suggested to increase the risk of Burnout. Although Maslach et al. (2001) argued that those who have obtained higher educational qualifications may be in jobs which have greater demands and expectations and therefore higher levels of stress, or alternatively those with higher levels of education have higher expectations for the careers they chose and therefore may experience more emotional distress if their expectations are not met. Freudenberger (1990) identified that therapists are often individuals who tend to exhibit higher expectations of themselves than of others and they focus on the needs of their clients whilst often neglecting to attend to their own needs which often results in them ignoring their own emotional distress.

Evidence concerning the complex relationship between gender and Burnout remains inconclusive. Some data has found no differences between it in different sexes (Carlson et al., 2003; Lemkau et al., 1987). Others indicate females experience higher Burnout levels than their male counterparts (McMurry et al., 2000; Cocco et al., 2003). Some studies have reported gender specific relationships between Burnout's individual components.

For example, Russell et al. (1987) and Schwab & Iwanicki (1982) found male teachers experienced higher levels of depersonalisation, whilst Maslach & Jackson (1985) found female health service professionals specifically experienced higher levels of emotional exhaustion and lower levels of personal accomplishment.

Martial status has also been examined and suggestions made that singles experienced higher Burnout levels than their married counterparts (Maslach et al., 2001; Gold, 1985). These authors also argue however there is insufficient empirical evidence for this relationship to be generalised and that the use of longitudinal studies may shed more light here.

The prevalence of the concept of Burnout appears to have been extensively researched over recent decades with studies covering those whose evidence is derived from field observations to the arena of systematic empirical reviews. The following studies are offered as a small sample of the diversity of occupation and geographical locations; air traffic controllers (Martinussen & Richardsen, 2006); U.S military nurses (Constable & Russell, 1986); German nursing staff (Bakker at al., 2000); Australian nursing staff (Rella et al., 2009); clergy (Rodgerson & Piedmont, 1998; Grosch & Olsen, 2000; Francis et al., 2004); doctors (Graham et al., 2000); general practitioners (Bakker et al., 2001); medical students in Sweden (Dahlin & Runeson, 2007); social workers (Acker & Lawrence, 2009) and teachers (Bakker & Schaufeil, 2000; Chan 2006).

In a valuable 12-year longitudinal study of young professionals Cherniss (1995) explored the professional journey of teachers, nurses, therapists and lawyers. This study was unusual on several fronts. Firstly, the duration of the study, as it allowed examination of professional journeys from their enthusiastic and idealistic conceptions to later stages, where individuals felt disillusioned. Additionally, the study was unique from a methodological standpoint as Cherniss sought the participant's free response narratives instead of providing a pre-determined list of responses from which participants select responses that appear to be the closest fit for their personal experience. The study's findings reported that positive experiences of autonomy, support and stimulation within the professional environment appeared to be factors that prevented Burnout.

In conclusion, this chapter has set out in detail the various concepts aligned with the negative impact of working with trauma. It has highlighted that evidence is emerging regarding the risks and impact of working with those who have experienced trauma (Pearlman & Mac Ian, 1995; Arvay, 2001; Figley, 2002a; Buchanan et al., 2006). However, it has also revealed that a number of diagnostic labels appear to have been assigned to the negative impact of trauma work and this has led to some confusion. Some studies deal with the concepts as being the same, some suggest they are related yet distinct and others ignore any association. It also revealed that several decades after the emergence of the idea that a professional may be impacted by their work with trauma, confusion remains around understanding the distinctiveness and relatedness of the various elements that comprise the secondary traumatisation experience (Harrison & Westwood, 2009; Figley, 2002a; Pearlman, 2003; Arvay, 2001).

This chapter has also highlighted that whilst the concepts share similarities in terms of risk and protective factors, the ways in which they manifest themselves are more distinct and potentially suggests it is not the diversity of concepts that has led to some confusion but the potential lack of clarification amongst researchers as to which of the particular concepts they are exploring and ensuring the appropriate measurement instruments are used.

It is the overlapping and at times interchangeable use of these terms that has potentially led to the confusion. The emphasis on quantitative methods over qualitative or mixed exploration of the concepts may have shown the 'what' of impact but evidence as to the 'how' or 'why' is much needed to fully understand the experience of working with trauma. Combining quantitative understandings with the personal accounts of those who live the experience will offer valuable insights into how numerical impact translates into real life emotions, thoughts and behaviours.

In moving forward, the following chapter will examine the literature specifically pertaining to the wider domain of clergy psychological wellbeing as it is essential to have a sound grasp of the current understanding of how faith leaders are functioning more generally before Chapter 5 moves to the crux of this book, to discuss the specific issue of the cost to clergy for caring for those who have experienced trauma and crisis.

Chapter 4

Clergy Psychological Wellbeing: The Wider Stresses of the Ministry

It has been argued that working in Christian ministry is a stressful process (Miner, 2007a). Empirical research indicates that clergy across religious orientations and geographic locations report poor work-related psychological health (Francis et al., 2004; Francis & Turton, 2004; Rutledge & Francis, 2004). This has resulted in the recognition that the issues of poor clergy psychological health and clergy burnout are increasingly prevalent problems (Lewis et al., 2007). Therefore, this chapter shall move beyond vicarious impact to examine the literature in relation to the wider concept of clergy psychological wellbeing.

Studies exploring work-related psychological health of the clergy have focused more prevalently on the final outcome of burnout (Francis et al., 2004; Rutledge & Francis, 2004; Randall, 2004; 2007; Raj & Dean, 2005; Doolittle, 2007; Miner, 2007a; Miner, 2007b; Turton & Francis, 2007; Chandler, 2009; Francis et al., 2009). However, the identification of secondary impact, which may potentially contribute to burnout, appears to have been overlooked. Indeed, when exploring factors which lead to clergy burnout, the issue of how the clergy are affected by their parishioners' trauma does not appear to be addressed, despite as Joinson (1992, p116) argues, that compassion fatigue may be a '*unique form*' of burnout.

The challenges of exploring any form of negative impact amongst clergy may be reflective of the influence of several elements. Firstly, Mc-Allister (1993) argues that religious professionals are often uncomfortable dealing with the negative emotions that are an associated part of their job as they, '*frequently have a sense of shame in having emotions which are not easily controlled*' (p216). This logic is supported by Grosch & Olsen (2000) examining clergy burnout from an integrative perspective. These authors suggest that for many parishioners the cleric is an idealisation of a father figure. Indeed, in some faiths he is even referred to as 'father' and this idealisation can result in the clergy striving to fulfil what may be the unrealistic expectations of their parishioners, through excessive workloads, not asking for help when needed and being totally at the beck and call of their parishioners with little thought for their own well-being. This mind-set and behaviour is carried out solely to produce what Grosch & Olsen (2000, p 622) refer to as "*a model of calmness, infallibility and perfection*". The ultimate result of this is a cleric who must work under increasing pressure to sustain this picture perfect. This would offer support for McAllister's (1993) argument that religious professionals are often uncomfortable dealing with the negative emotions, which are an associated part of their job.

Considering this argument, it may be logical to assume that the clergy may have in the past been reticent to open up regarding this negative aspect of their ministry. This argument is further reinforced by Holaday et al.'s (2001) study; in the words of an American pastor who had been in the ministry for twenty years referring to discussing the problems associated with pastoral counselling, *'We don't talk about these things at conferences. I have never talked about this before and it's important'* (p57). This reticence regarding discussion on the part of the clergy may in turn have led others to assume that either they are not undergoing negative experiences, or if they are, they are not willing to make the experience known. The lack of willingness to acknowledge they are negatively impacted may have resulted in the adoption of a *'walking on water syndrome'*, i.e., failing to recognise or accept one's own humanity and vulnerability (Holaday et al., 2001). By adopting this approach some clergy may be placing themselves in a precarious position regarding recognising, acknowledging and managing these issues. However, thankfully it would appear that the tide is turning and emerging research is now permitting us to glimpse that the clergy, like other populations, are subjected to negative experiences in the course of their work resulting in stress and burnout (Darling et al., 2004; Lee, 2007; Francis et al., 2008; Charlton et al., 2009).

Kinman et al. (2011) examined the cost to clergy in relation to Hochschild's concept of 'emotional labour (1983) which is viewed as being required to exhibit organisationally accepted emotions within interpersonal encounters. Findings suggested that there were clearly costs to clergy when they perceived a dissonance between the emotions they were expected to display and those they felt would be acceptable. Hendron (2013) also referred to this with clergy recalling how at times they were at odds with their perceived requirements of their role. For example, being the calm presence within a parishioner's crisis storm could be a world away from the emotions they were feeling and the sheer effort of managing these emotional displays to meet role requirements was often exhausting.

Early exit from the ministry is an increasing problem (Beebe, 2007) and yet this is hardly surprising given the work of the Christian ministry is frequently portrayed as a stressful vocation which is conductive to the experience of burnout (Sanford,1982; Croucher, 1991; Kaldor & Bullpitt, 2001; Miner, 2007a).

In relation to pastoral burnout, researchers have attempted to examine some of the issues that specifically affect this population. These include, but are not exclusive to, the impact of rest, support and spiritual renewal (Chandler, 2009); burnout and depression (Raj & Dean, 2005); burnout and coping in parish ministry (Doolittle, 2007) burnout during the first twelve months of ministry (Miner, 2007a, 2007b); burnout and prayer (Turton & Francis, 2007), burnout amongst Roman Catholic clergy (Francis et al., 2004); burnout amongst Anglican male clergy (Rutledge & Francis, 2004); burnout amongst Australian clergy (Francis et al., 2009).

Miner (2007a) examined the views of clergy on whether work or personal issues were more stressful in the twelve months post-graduation, exploring if these stressors were related to burnout. She also examined 'personal factors' which had previously been aligned with burnout in previous studies; age (Francis & Rutledge,

2000; Francis et al., 2004; Randall, 2004) personality traits (Francis et al., 2004; Hills et al., 2004) and religious coping styles (Rodgerson & Piedmont, 1998). Her findings indicated relational and ministry issues were found to cause most stress over the first twelve months period. Miner's (2007a) findings made no mention by participants of any stress associated with working with individuals who had traumatic material, although this may have been alluded to in the mention of the parishioners' needs and losses being stressful situations over which the clergy felt they had little control.

Additional studies have highlighted that during their first year post theological training the majority of ministers reported relational and ministry issues to be most severe and contributing to their overall stress in a significant way, (Whetham & Whetham, 2000; Milner, 2007b). Additionally, links have emerged between age and clergy burnout (Kaldor & Bullpitt, 2001; Roberts et al., 2003; Francis et al., 2004; Randall, 2004). In light of the identification of lack of experience and youth as being potential risk factors for secondary traumatisation (Marmar et al., 1996; Resick, 2000; Adams et al., 2001), these studies, which align lack of experience and youth with burnout, must be considered as being of potential relevance to the understanding of secondary traumatisation amongst clergy.

Conversly, Hendron (2013) found increased years in ministry was associated with higher levels of secondary traumatic stress. Interviews revealed that this might be due to several factors. Participants often recalled the three-year period post ordination as the "golden years". This was due to the fact clerics new to the role were in curate positions and therefore felt generally supported by their more experienced superiors. This situation appeared to change dramatically once the role of curate became that of a fist time rector. At this juncture participants reported feeling that support diminished and stress increased and relationships with parishioners became much more blurred as strong friendships developed over sustained periods of time.

Some studies have indicated no significant difference between clergy and non-clergy burnout scores (Warner & Carter, 1984). However, the results of that study were interesting in that clergy wives scored highest on the burnout dimension of emotional exhaustion. Virginia (1998) reported that secular Roman Catholic clergy had higher levels of emotional exhaustion, depression and burnout than their counterparts in religious orders and monastic locations. Spencer et al. (2012) attempted to predict levels of risk for a pastor within their role and here the issues of ministerial expectation versus ministerial realities were exposed. To capture concepts that portrayed a sense of failure derived from unrealistic expectation the authors coined the term *'vision conflict'* and to capture concepts reflecting the overwhelming physical and emotional demands of the ministry they applied the term *'compassion fatigue'* (p 88). These authors made no mention of trauma involvement and reported compassion fatigue was significantly different between clergy working in churches where previous rectors had been forced to resign and those who were not in this situation. Compassion fatigue was also related to having no regular support and congregational attendances that remained static or declined.

Berry et al. (2012) adopted an insightful approach to clergy burnout through employing qualitative methods to explore ministry and stress amongst Anglican clergy in Wales. The study presented themes relating to personal assessment of their health, assessing causes and symptoms of stress, naming support, forms of relaxation and enhancing clergy training. These authors reported this sample of clergy appeared to be indicating signs of overwork but they were engaged with the impact of their ministry and were aware of the signs of stress. The authors also highlighted the need for those responsible for clergy welfare to take note of the accounts given and to recognise the demands of ministry.

This chapter has focused on the wider area of clergy wellbeing. This has revealed several key points. Firstly, it suggests that many clerics find their role to be a challenging one and that this often demands a cost in terms of their physical and mental wellbeing. The chapter also revealed that whilst valuable work has been undertaken within the domain of clergy burnout the consequences of working with trauma have not really been considered extensively as potential factors on the road to early exit from the ministry. Therefore, the focus of the following chapter will be the impact upon clergy from specifically working with trauma and crisis within their Pastoral Ministry.

Chapter 5

When Caring Hurts: Impact upon Clergy when Working with Crisis

This chapter deals with the very crux of this book in that it sets out the small but significant body of research which focuses specifically on what is known regarding clergy and vicarious impact. The preceding discussions have highlighted that those involved in the care of individuals and communities who have experienced tragedy are at risk of experiencing some level of impact simply from their involvement (McCann & Pearlman, 1990a; Figley,1995; Stamm, 2009). Lerias & Byrne (2003) defined a vicarious impact reaction as:

> *"The response of those persons who have witnessed, been subject to explicit knowledge of, or had the responsibility to intervene in a seriously distressing or tragic event".* (p130).

Furthermore, these authors identify this impact as a natural consequence stemming from the care that individuals provide. When such a suggestion is aligned with clergy involvement with human tragedy either directly or vicariously through their pastoral ministry, then we should hardly be surprised that for some, or perhaps many, the impact from their work can and does resonate within both their professional and personal lives.

To recap, previous discussions in this book have highlighted the work of the Pastoral Ministry, identified that clergy are frequently at the coalface within communities and that clergy are at risk of diminished psychological wellbeing.

However, previous chapters have focused on the more general areas of clergy stress and burnout. To present a comprehensive understanding of the situation for clergy in relation to vicarious impact from trauma work this chapter will encompass the wide spectrum of work ranging from major trauma incidents to those smaller scale incidences that form a key part of the pastoral ministry. This is all undertaken to make the point that many clergy may well be at risk of secondary trauma from the greater and lesser demands the pastoral element of their role places upon them.

Clergy have often been involved in major trauma events either individually or as part of larger trauma response teams. Events that unfolded in New York on September 11th, 2001, as the Twin Towers and the city of New York came under terrorist attack, temporarily focused the lens of secondary impact research in part upon clergy trauma work. Roberts et al. (2003) examined compassion fatigue amongst chaplains, clergy and other respondents after 9/11. Clergy participants made up 78.5% of the study's sample with the rest being made up from mental health practitioners, seminary students, executives from mental health and disaster relief agencies and other individuals who provided direct relief services. Roberts et al. (2003) reported that a large portion of their sample were at significant risk of compassion fatigue (27.5% = extremely high, 11.7 = high risk). The only variable found to be significantly associated with compassion fatigue was whether a participant worked as part of a relief agency such as the American Red Cross. Roberts et al. (2003) claimed that a substantial proportion of the clergy in the Tri-State area were at significant risk for compassion fatigue and the mean risk for compassion fatigue and burnout for the entire sample was higher than that of the validation sample for the test. Although this sample did not consist of 100% clergy, nevertheless the numbers of clergy involved do make it valuable in directing attention toward the fact that clergy are at risk of secondary impact through the very nature of their work. Furthermore, it offers confirmation that during the events of 9/11 the clergy served as frontline workers within their communities.

Flannelly et al. (2005) focused solely on clergy participants with a total of 342 clergy including 149 (43.4%) who acted as disaster relief workers after the 9/11 attacks. Those who worked as part of a disaster agency such as The American Red Cross were labelled 'responders' in contrast to those who were not involved with a disaster agency who were labelled as 'non-responders'. Therefore, from the outset one can clearly see the value of this study in that it afforded an opportunity to compare impact between these groups. Employing the Compassion Satisfaction and Fatigue Test (Figley, 1995), their findings provided valuable insights into what took place in the lives of these individuals.

Amongst non-responders, being a chaplain and the number of hours worked with trauma victims were positively related to compassion fatigue. Having undertaken Clinical Pastoral Education was inversely related to compassion fatigue, whilst amongst responders the hours worked with trauma victims was significantly related to compassion fatigue. The number of days spent at Ground Zero also made a significant difference to levels of compassion fatigue. Results highlighted the potential benefits of training and support in that impact levels were lower amongst those who had worked with The American Red Cross. In fact, responders who worked with this agency reported lower levels of impact than non-responders, whilst responders who had not worked within its framework reported higher levels of impact than non-responders. The overall suggestion of the study was that clergy played an important part in the events of 9/11 and increased exposure to these events increased compassion fatigue. Additionally, training and support from an agency such as the American Red Cross that has expertise in disaster work was shown to be beneficial.

Quite understandably, given its history of violence, the involvement of Northern Ireland's clergy in the troubles has been explored. Gibson & Iwaniec (2003) examined professionals involved in the aftermath of two specific trauma events. Whilst not solely focusing on a clergy sample their participants did include clergy who had been involved in caring for those impacted by the Shankill bombing on 23rd October 1993 when the Irish Republican Army detonated a bomb in a shop situated in a busy area in Belfast. The no warning bomb caused the death of 10 people and injured around 52 others. Clergy involved in the study indicated that this was not their first traumatic event and that they dealt on a continual basis with their traumatised communities. Clergy participants indicated they had received training in pastoral care, but none had received any training on how to cope with their personal reactions to their work.

There have also been several studies involving clergy and trauma work that focus less on major trauma events. In 2001, one of the first studies focusing specifically on clergy and the area of secondary impact was undertaken by Holaday and colleagues. These researchers adopted a mixed methodology to examine secondary impact amongst a sample of 30 male and female American pastors. There was a very specific focus within this study as these pastors were identified as those who specifically provided counselling as part of their religious duties.

Given that much of the vicarious impact research was at that time based upon those within the counselling and psychotherapy professions, Holaday et al (2001) had a justification for the specificity of their study. Clergy participants completed several recognised measurement instruments; The Maslach Burnout inventory, (MBI), (Maslach & Jackson, 1986), which is used to measure burnout through the three dimensions of emotional exhaustion, depersonalisation and personal accomplishment and the Traumatic Stress Institute Belief Scale (Traumatic Stress Institute, 1997), an instrument designed to measure disrupted cognitive schemas in the five psychological needs areas of safety, trust, control, intimacy and esteem. In addition to revealing levels of impact the study also reported several areas of interest including the costs of listening to problems and coping strategies used to handle the stress of the encounters and advice for new clergy.

One highly valuable aspect of this study was the employment of a mixed methods approach gleaning both numerical and narrative data. It revealed key insights into how this sample of clergy appeared to be willing to discuss issues verbally but appeared less willing to commit their comments to paper.

Comparison of clergy scores on the Belief Scale with scores from mental health professionals and students revealed that clergy had experienced impact that caused cognitive disruptions. Using the scales normative data clergy totals were higher than mental health professionals but lower than student samples (clergy=181.60, mental health professionals=166.83, students=192.41). In relation to burnout, results for the MBI indicated 57% of clergy had moderate to high scores on the emotional exhaustion component, 35% reported moderate/high scores on depersonalisation and 97% moderate/high scores on the personal accomplishment subscale. Total Belief scores significantly correlated with the Emotional Exhaustion subscale of the MBI leading the authors to suggest that these scales measure related yet separate constructs. However, the authors did not appear to consider the possibility that this correlation could be due in part to the disruptions recorded by the Belief Scale feeding into and elevating levels of emotional exhaustion. They also reported correlations between high scores in emotional exhaustion and high scores in self/other trust, leading them to posit that when under stress, clergy have difficulty in trusting judgments made by themselves or others and consequently they feel they cannot rely on others to meet their psychological needs. These findings support other studies amongst other professions that have reported a disruption in trust due to vicarious exposure to trauma (Pearlman & Mac-Ian, 1995; Schauben & Frazer, 1995; Arvay & Uhlemann, 1996; Steed & Dowling, 1998; Black & Weinreich, 2001).

The qualitative aspect of their study revealed most of the clergy interviewed encountered emotional and physical strain in relation to dealing with individuals who had experienced a range of issues including sexual abuse, suicidal thoughts, mental and terminal illnesses. The authors concluded that, clergy are exposed to traumatic material, similar in content to that encountered by their counterparts within other caring professions.

The experience of dealing with illness and death in children was identified as being one of the most difficult, with one cleric reporting it caused feelings of total helplessness which left him feeling unable to discuss this experience even with his spouse. Barnsteiner & Gilles-Donovan (1990) suggested that life-threatening illness in children creates powerful emotions and those who work with vulnerable populations such as ill and dying children have been identified as being at higher risk of secondary traumatisation (Beaton & Murphy, 1995).

In relation to more interpersonal and community events, Hendron (2013) sheds further light on the experiences of and the impact upon clergy. Employing both quantitative and qualitative methods this study explored the experience of vicarious impact within the pastoral ministry of 226 clergy based across Ireland. In relation to levels of impact all 226 participants recorded some level of impact as measured by the Secondary Traumatic Stress subscale on the ProQOL V (Stamm, 2009), with almost a third falling within the higher range of scores. This suggests that involvement in crisis related situations within the pastoral ministry has the potential to evoke a negative impact. In addition to being of empirical interest, this finding should be a major concern to both individual clergy and those with a remit for their care as it demonstrates there is a high emotional and psychological cost being paid for this aspect of the pastoral ministry.

Qualitative interviews in this study shed further light on the situation. One might assume that scores of this nature would indicate individuals who were broken men and women but on the contrary, many participants appeared to have become masters at putting on displays of normality so that few others, apart from their closest family, recognise the high price they pay in terms of their physical, cognitive and emotional wellbeing. Participants within Hendron's study also stated that within these traumas there was the expectation they would have the professional knowledge and spiritual answers to deal with diverse issues, ranging from martial disputes to helping a family through the aftermath of suicide. It became clear their trauma work is compounded by feelings of pressure to provide spiritual and secular solutions for the tragic events that have occurred. This subject has surfaced before within the literature with a sample of American clergy speaking of being expected to '*have the answers*' and '*make things better for people*" and "*I used to feel that it was my responsibility to take care of people*' (Holaday et al., 2001, p59).

Hendron explored the issues that clergy identified as being the most traumatic to deal with. Hardly surprisingly bereavement and terminal illness are two of the most commonly experienced issues with participants stating death as the issue they find the most difficult to deal with. This finding concurs with prior literature reporting bereavement and illness issues are the most common problems clergy face (Wright, 1984; Lount & Hargie, 1997; Francis et al., 2000; Flannelly et al., 2003; Turton, 2010). Hendron (2013) also highlighted a disturbing catalogue of challenging experiences clergy are involved with including issues such as domestic violence, man-made atrocities, sexual abuse, supporting survivors of the Northern Ireland troubles, natural disasters, on-going international wars and economic downturns. Many identified their knowledge of dealing with issues such as suicide, murder, dementia and increasing natural disasters such as flooding, fell well outside their range of expertise and training, yet they could not walk away from them.

The previous studies discussed have already identified that clerics are frequently part of the first responder team. Hendron (2013) found numerous clergy accounts of parishioners accessing them as a first port of call when a crisis occurs and in some cases, they are accessed by those who have previously had little or no contact with a faith community. This supports the proposal by Meek et al. (2003) that "for *these people the clergy person is and always will be, the therapist on call*". Clearly clergy are not merely being accessed as carers of souls but are being accessed by individuals and communities for a range of issues resulting in them taking on the guise of pseudo counsellors, social workers and mental health therapists. This adds weight to Switzer's (2000) argument that the types of issues brought to the clergy are as wide ranging as the human predicament and are often because of crisis situations. This supports prior arguments that clergy are often the first accessed means of support for many individuals (Weaver et al., 2003; Oppenheimer et al., 2004; Hendron et al., 2012).

Hendron's (2013) findings also offer support for the arguments of Wang et al. (2003) who suggest the work of 21st century clergy is spreading beyond spiritual support and infiltrating the worlds of mental health professionals and counsellors. Indeed, there are clear indicators clergy are potentially having more diverse and more difficult 'case loads' than they may have had even a decade ago.

These findings clearly indicate several key points. Firstly, the need for clergy training to stay abreast of current societal issues to ensure those sent out to undertake this role are equipped not for a by gone era but for the realities of 21st century ministry. It also suggests clergy should be recognised within the wider sphere of health professionals as a valuable community resource in line with arguments raised by other authors, (Weaver et al., 1996; O'Kane & Millar, 2001; Oppenheimer et al., 2004; Leavey et al., 2007).

The issue of expectations weighing heavily upon clergy shoulders is not a new one, although it is more historically aligned with general stress and burnout than adding pressure to the secondary traumatisation experience. Barna (1999, p37) suggested many churches pressurise their pastors through expecting them to be "*masters of all trades*" and these "*unrealistic expectations*" help to explain why clergy stress incidences have grown to dangerous proportions. This conversation is important as it provides evidence that the issue of expectations transfers into this element of the clergy role and as such, potentially needs addressed during training and through on-going support.

Chaplains are also of specific interest in that by its very nature the chaplain role involves individual and community crisis work. Galek et al. (2011) examined the extent to which work related and social support variables predicted vicarious impact amongst 331 chaplains. One of this study's great strengths lay within its sample which comprised a diverse range of theological orientations (67.7% Protestant, 25.7% Catholic and 5.7% Jewish) working as chaplains and that it tried to distinguish the concepts of secondary traumatic stress and burnout as being separate yet related. Results indicated secondary traumatic stress levels but not burnout levels were positively associated with hours worked with trauma clients. Chaplains working within hospital settings were not found to be more susceptible to secondary traumatic stress despite having more potential exposure to traumatised individuals. Additionally, years of experience were not related to secondary traumatic stress but were related to burnout. Whilst the authors did not elaborate these findings, they may suggest that as hospital chaplains encounter individuals whom they have no prior relationship or knowledge of, they may be in a better position to remain emotionally removed from what is taking place.

How vicarious impact reveals its symptoms within lives is important as quite naturally it is one thing to report a high score on a validated scale but understanding how these scores translate into everyday personal and professional lives merits explanation. The qualitative element of Hendron's (2013) study provided valuable insights into this with those who scored highest in secondary traumatic stress giving accounts of the severest physical, emotional and behavioural symptoms. Some recalled extreme behaviours impacting their personal lives through illness, fatigue and depression, their professional lives through altered relationships with parishioners and their family lives through developments of bizarre behaviours. Whilst disruptions to the professional's family are sometimes an indicator that all is not well, disruptions have previously been reported as 'unavailability' for the family, in terms of being unable to give attention or being too busy with work (Ben-Porat & Itzhaky, 2009). The taking of active steps to remove themselves emotionally and physically from their parishioners, especially when this removal comes at the cost to their family, takes 'unavailability' to another level and indicates the severity of the situation for some participants.

Figley (1995) suggests symptoms of vicarious impact often mimic those of Post-Traumatic Stress Disorder, (PTSD), therefore this behaviour is suggestive of the 'avoidance' element of this condition. Other participants spoke of re-experiencing accounts of trauma they had been involved in and especially those that involved terrorist incidents. Once again this is in line with secondary trauma symptoms mimicking those of PTSD with accounts of flashbacks and nightmares. However, for some, re-experiencing involves not only the event itself but also a reminder of their helplessness to avoid the situation. For some this work appears to have left what Hendron (2013) termed a 'sacred scar', as clergy joyfully bear as part of their calling to undertake Christ's ministry here on earth. Others appeared less affected by the work, although deeper conversations revealed this appears to be a result of emotional and physical distancing at times between these clergy and those they care for. Whilst this has protected them from the severest impact it potentially has repercussions within their wider ministries.

Hendron (2013) stated that cognitive/emotional disruptions were especially painful to observe as they painted a portrait of individuals whose self-esteem, belief and trust in themselves and others appears to have been eroded through this element of their pastoral work. Alterations in self-esteem were also observed. McCann & Pearlman (1990a) propose self-esteem can be defined as '*the belief in one's value*'. When we have a positive view of ourselves we are more likely to have a positive view of others. Trauma exposure can cause alterations in our view of our self and this alteration often manifests itself in a distorted and cynical conception of others. Hendron (2013) illustrated this altered view of the self in the painfully articulated and despairing words of a participant: "*I disappeared*'.

McCann & Pearlman's (1990a) Constructivist Self Development Theory as previously discussed in Chapter Three is of value here as it postulates the concept of 'self' as central to everyone's worldview. According to these authors the 'self' we think we are, is formed through personal experiences and interpretations of the world. This 'self' in turn defines the meanings we attribute to and gain from life. Therefore, development of 'self' is a fragile evolving process that can be damaged by life experiences.

Sadly, accounts of suicidal thoughts amongst clergy have previously been revealed. Turton (2010) examined mental health in clergy and recorded 21% of his participants had experienced acute anxiety; 30% depression; 3% nervous breakdown and 8% suicidal thoughts. Whilst Hendron (2013) acknowledges that the challenges of the pastoral ministry element of their work may not be the only factor that has led some participants to feel this way, her findings did imply involvement in crisis and trauma work does appear to severely impact some individuals and it may be when combined with other personal or professional difficulties the situation becomes untenable.

Given that clerics are feeling impacted, questions need to be asked regarding the spread of ripples from this impact beyond the cleric. The idea that a negative impact from the ministry can invade the lives of those directly connected with clergy is no new thing and has previously been identified within the more general domain of clergy stress (Darling et al., 2004; Lee, 2007; Burton & Burton, 2009) and in relation to rectory families being placed under more intense public scrutiny and expectations of certain behaviours (Finch, 1983).

Although not focusing on trauma work, Darling et al. (2004) examined stress and quality of life for clergy and their spouses. They reported spouses were at as high a risk as clergy for moderate to extremely high levels of compassion fatigue (clergy 26.9%, spouses 26.5%) and moderate to extremely high potential for burnout (clergy 22%, spouses 20.5%). Spouses reported lower potential for satisfaction in their role compared to clergy (spouses 52.1%, clergy 28.6 %). These findings indicate the emotional demands of the clergy role resonate within the spousal role and may allude to the existence of tertiary trauma.

Hendron's (2013) work is useful for this in that it suggested that there may be an experience of tertiary trauma for those who care for the carers, with accounts of wives and peers experiencing signs of secondary trauma impact through their third hand exposure. Some of these participants felt they were spreading impact beyond themselves to others and this in turn had spun a web of guilt and frustration.

Within the secondary trauma literature, emotional contagion to family members is discussed in the form of primary trauma 'contaminating' family members through contact (Figley, 1983). In these situations, the family member rather than the professional is the vicarious observer of the initial trauma. A few studies have explored this aspect of vicarious exposure within family members of: combat veterans (Scaturo & Hayman, 1992) and children of parents with mental illness (Lombardo & Motta, 2008). Regehr (2005) indicated paramedics' family members were impacted by their work although this impact was described in terms of the paramedics emotionally distancing themselves from families or their displays of anger or irritability with family members.

How does peer support fit within this puzzle given that amongst other caring professions peer support is often seen as a common method for dealing with vicarious impact? Pearlman & Mac Ian (1993) reported 85% of their sample of trauma counsellors use peers as the most common method for dealing with the effects of vicarious trauma. Peer sharing has been viewed as a healthy outlet (Pearlman & Saakvitne, 1995a) and hailed as a powerful factor in the prevention and amelioration of secondary impact.

Many authors paint an equally rosy picture of peer sharing (Kassen-Adams, 1995; Avery & Uhleman, 1996; Rudolph & Stamm, 1999; Adams et al., 2001; Bober & Regehr, 2006). For example, Catherall (1995) contends peer supervision groups serve as important resources amongst trauma counsellors whilst Dyregrov & Mitchell (1996) suggested talking with co-workers about trauma responses offered valuable support in dealing with the after effects of the work. Saakvitne & Pearlman (1996) resonate this call stating colleagues form an important part of self-care, advocating that colleagues can be a lifeline for sharing work difficulties because they not only understand the work, but also understand issues surrounding confidentiality.

The emergence of these positive conversations regarding peer support may be reflective of contrasts between clergy and other professions that offer superior training and support to that found amongst clergy and as such, peers in these professions are better equipped to help each other. Potentially the mental health environment that prompted original suggestions of peer support as a protective factor, offers individuals the tools to manage their own impact and thus better equips them to assist each other go through similar experiences without being diminished themselves.

Hendron (2013) also revealed that the peer support experiences for some is not a positive occurrence and those who provide informal peer support can feel negative effects similar to those they try to help. This draws important attention to the fact that whilst the 'peer sharing' process may be a positive experience for those seeking to share, for the other party involved, it can be a toxic experience. Such issues raise serious implications for individual clergy but also for their spouses, their peers and those with a duty of care towards these individuals. Church organisations need to ensure that adequate formal support is provided in an effort to reduce the need to share informally with those who are ill prepared to handle the experience.

As discussed in previous chapters, the concept of spirituality has been associated both as a protective factor and as an aspect of the individual that can be damaged by association with the trauma (Saakvitne & Pearlman, 1996) and stress emerging from life's challenges, such as job-related stress (Csiernik & Adams, 2002) and health related stress (Jenkins & Pargament, 1995; Bulman & Wortman, 1997; Siegel et al., 2001). Oman & Thoresen (2005) contend there is growing evidence that a connection with religion or spirituality is associated with enhanced physical and mental wellbeing and spiritual resources have also been linked to physical and mental health (Genia & Shaw, 1991; Koenig et al., 2001; Joshi et al., 2008). Given these prior associations and assumptions, the value of being able to explore the influence of secondary impact upon spirituality within a highly spiritual group is very significant.

Hendron (2013) afforded a unique examination of this aspect of secondary impact within a religious profession and results indicated that given all 226 participants reported some level of impact, spirituality would not appear to be a 'cloak of invisibility' which one can put on to avoid being affected by this work. Interviews facilitated further exploration of spirituality within this experience and extreme care was taken within discussions to avoid the specific use of the term 'spirituality', as if mentioned, participants might have felt implicit pressures to report positively in relation to this topic. In an attempt not to lead or pressurise participants the topic was explored through the question '*Is there anything which protects you or makes you vulnerable in this experience*?' presupposing that this question could offer participants an opportunity to discuss the role their faith had played.

Surprisingly, in some interviews the subject of God or faith was not mentioned. This could be construed as the result of several different mindsets. Firstly, it could indicate that given their clergy role, participants assumed their acceptance of the influence of their faith would be assumed and therefore there was no need to mention it. Secondly, these individuals, whose personal and profession essence is so intrinsically tied to their faith and spirituality, felt under pressure not to admit a cost that involved their spirituality. However, given their honesty in other aspects of the interviews the researcher did not believe participants intentionally held back on this subject.

Amongst those who did address the subject there was no mention of their faith in God being altered and for some their faith appeared to have been strengthened through the challenges presented by this work. This finding is reflective of an older study by Brady et al. (1999) who reported that clinicians who had large caseloads of sexual abuse survivors indicated that their spirituality was actually increased rather than damaged by their vicarious exposure to clients' trauma.

What did emerge was an understanding that their belief in God's people had been shaken. This appeared to cause certain problems and some who mentioned their shattered assumptions that God's people would be supportive and caring, also went on to speak about conflicts with parishioners and vestries, suggesting this strand of impact had far reaching effects within their wider ministry. There are clear implications here for training in that care needs to be taken when presenting the concept of spirituality as protective against secondary impact within training, particularly amongst faith groups. Presenting spirituality too strongly as a protective factor could result in those who experience impact and who have a faith, not admitting impact or seeking help due to fear of their actions being perceived as a lack of faith.

Exposure to trauma appears to be made more difficult for clergy through the complexities of the relationships they have with those they care for. For some this takes the form of knowing those involved prior to a crisis event taking place. Hendron (2013) found that this appeared to evoke an emotional involvement with those they care for resulting in clergy finding it hard to remain the objective professional. Some even mentioned how at times they feel God sends them a death of someone they do not know or had no long-term involvement with as a means of relief.

There appear to have been no studies that directly explore secondary trauma amongst those who have a prior relationship with the primary victim. The closest study found to this topic was by Feldman & Kaal (2007) who were not seeking to explicitly explore levels of impact amongst those who had prior relationships with victims but who focused on alterations in world assumptive views (Janoff-Bulman, 1985). Their findings reported secondary exposure alone was not associated with a negative assumptive worldview, but it was the combination of a relationship with victims along with higher levels of empathy that was related to less belief in a meaningful world.

In a more recent study, oncology nurses reported that at times they became emotionally involved with patients and their families which they believed increased their risk of feeling an impact from their work (Perry et al., 2011). Hendron's (2013) study involved some revealing conversations that started to explore the differences in secondary impact when personal/professional boundaries are blurred and this is an area that requires further exploration.

A further component of exposure complexity is the long-term contact clergy have with those affected. This appeared to follow on naturally from the previous topic of prior relationships with direct victims of trauma. There were frequent referrals to being on a 'journey' with those they care for. Accounts emerged of feeling re-traumatised through ministering sometimes over periods of many years to individuals who were the primary victims.

Once again this is a factor not addressed within the secondary trauma literature and as with the previous topic it is one that may well not have appeared before due to the fact that within many professions the blurring of professional and personal boundaries would be frowned upon.

In professions such as counselling, the professional framework does not normally advocate working with individuals who are personally know to the professional and they would not encourage any on-going contact once therapy had ended (McLeod, 2003). Yet the clergy role is one in which a personal on-going relationship with parishioners is an integral part of the role and as such potentially increases the cleric's vulnerability to secondary impact. Leavey et al. (2007) touched upon this subject but from the standpoint of parishioners rather than the clergy, suggesting the close relationships priests had with their parishioners fostered the growth of pastoral support. When Leavey et al.'s finding is aligned with Hendron (2013), it would suggest what may be beneficial for parishioners could at times demand a cost from the clerics.

Part of the fundamental problem here may stem back to a lack of a clearly defined role for clergy. Miner (1992) contends role ambiguity occurs when role related information is not available. Give that clergy mentioned they have no clear job descriptions and decisions as to what is included and excluded in the role are often left up to the individual as there are no professional guidelines on maintaining boundaries. Role ambiguity is not a new problem for clergy although it has previously been associated with general stress levels (Hang-yue et al., 2005; Kemery, 2006).

The combination of long term involvement and blurred relationships suggests some clergy may be at risk of secondary trauma more from the stance of a family member rather than that of a professional. Secondary impact has been identified within family relationships; children of Vietnam veterans (Motta et al., 1997; Suozzia & Motta, 2004); wives of veterans with PTSD (Waysman et al., 1993); post generations of Holocaust survivors (Kassai & Motta, 2006); family members of those suffering serious illness (Boyer et al., 2000; Lombardo & Motta, 2008). Therefore, more research is needed to fully understand the influence these complex factors have upon the secondary traumatisation experience in order to customise training and support for clergy in this work.

Working with crisis is only one aspect of the pastoral ministry and the clergy role involves other positive elements such as teaching, baptisms, marriages and preaching (Darling et al., 2004). Therefore, one would instinctively expect the more positive aspects of the ministry to act as counterbalances for the negative aspects. However, Hendron (2013) found indications that being able to deal with the extremes of human life within the space of a day can for some be a source of difficulty and strain rather than a source of satisfaction.

This echoes Kinman et al.'s (2011) suggestion that when clergy are under pressure to display organisationally acceptable emotional responses, they are more likely to experience psychological distress. It also builds on knowledge provided by Turton (2010) who discussed the demands of dealing with such extremes and proposed clergy were often involved in several situations within a short space of time, which require dramatic changes in their attitudes and self-awareness. These demands he suggests are not normally expected within other professions but do impact clergy. Hendron (2013) found some participants indicating that being able to switch emotions quickly as they moved between the very positive aspects of the ministry to the negative aspects often within a very short timescale rather than alleviating pressure, actually increased it. Hochschild's (1983) concept of emotional labour is also worth revisiting at this point. It has been previously examined within Chapter 4 however, in light of the discussions that have just taken place, then clergy should be made aware that at times what they feel and how professionally they are expected to behave may be vastly different. This naturally may result in stressors that they will need to be aware of, recognise and explore positive ways to manage this.

Weaver et al. (2003) suggest that the frequency with which clergy are accessed during times of crisis is due in part to their availability. Hendron (2013) showed this availability may be good news for those they help but less so for clergy themselves. The challenges of managing their availability to these events and the stresses caused by parishioners being able to contact them at any time of the day or night is a cause for concern. This situation is compounded by the fact their place of work is also their home. Clergy inability to regulate and control their exposure and not being able to resolve one issue before being confronted by the next is entwined with feelings of guilt and frustration. Once again this is perhaps an issue not seen within other professions that have clear lines of demarcation between places of work and home.

As previously mentioned the inability to maintain boundaries is not a new problem for clergy. Russell (1984) suggests this practice emerged from the Victorian era where the notion existed that the professional was never off duty, resulting in blurred boundaries between personal and professional time. This is potentially one of the most difficult aspects for clergy to realistically manage. Hendron (2013) reported that some participants with low levels of secondary traumatic stress indicated they did not encourage an 'open all hours' policy, although this could have a detrimental effect on their wider ministry.

In order to overcome this problem, it may be valuable to promote good self-care strategies amongst clergy that embrace the concepts of adequate time off as essential rather than optional. It may also be beneficial to educate those involved with clergy at vestry and parishioner level and encourage these individuals to take responsibility for the welfare of their cleric through accepting personal space and time off as necessary components of the ministry.

The term 'pri-sec' trauma was coined by Hendron (2013), in an attempt to capture the dual experiences of exposure to elements of primary and vicarious trauma, through on-going care for victims or survivors. Pri-sec exposure appears to take three forms:

- Being present at the actual event (e.g., being at a hospital when a child dies).

- Being involved with the immediate aftermath of the event (e.g., being there before the body was cut down in a suicide or present directly after bomb explosions).

- Direct trauma against clergy themselves (e.g., physically assaulted in the course of their work).

The early involvement in crisis situations seems to be a culture fostered amongst clergy right from the early days of their theological training. Hemmelgarn et al.

(2006) define the term *'organisational culture'* as the modelled and observed organisational norms, beliefs, and expectations that are inculcated in staff. Hendron (2013) suggests these norms and expectations are set in motion during theological training and whilst they may be beneficial for the ministry they can be potentially less beneficial for the cleric. However, they are recognised as an important aspect of the clergy role that, given societal expectations, would be unrealistic to change. Therefore, if this organisational ethos is encouraged, there must be adequate support in place such as critical incident debriefing (CID), in order to help clergy who are involved in events such as major terrorist incidents or road traffic accidents, to access a safe supportive environment in order to help them process and assimilate their experiences.

Hardly surprisingly involvement in the actual event or the immediate aftermath appears to result in increased absorption of the experience. So much so that some of Hendron's participants appeared to almost take on the realities of the parishioners' experiences as their own. Conrad & Gellar-Guenther (2006) contend the experience of secondary trauma is increased for the professional when they empathically enter the victim's world. This being the case, how much more problematic must it be for clergy who enter the world of the victim both vicariously through empathy and compassion and directly through physical contact.

From a fundamental vicarious impact standpoint, the emergence of this suggests levels of secondary trauma reported by some clergy may well be capturing some level of primary trauma as well. Given that Figley (1995) suggests secondary trauma symptoms often mimic those of primary trauma, it is not surprising the ProQOLV instrument used in Hendron's (2013) study picked up and combined both experiences. Once again this is a factor not explored within much of the literature although Flannelly et al. (2005) touched upon this without expanding the concept. They reported hours worked by clergy directly at Ground Zero was related to increased levels of compassion fatigue, suggesting it may well have been the sights and sounds of Ground Zero such as retrieving dead bodies that increased compassion satisfaction levels. Had Flannelly et al. (2005) delved deeper into the merging of the worlds of victims and helpers then potentially some precious insights could have been gleaned into this unusual element of trauma work.

White (2001) also touched upon this subject discussing the dual experience of being personally affected by an event as well as providing care to others who are affected, although this was from the standpoint of therapists who lived and worked near Ground Zero and were themselves directly impacted by the events of 9/11 in addition to caring for its survivors.

Hendron (2013) reported a key finding in relation to length of service increasing negative impact. This was extremely important in that it was atypical to the existing literature on secondary impact, that suggests the risk is normally higher for those who are new to their roles. Quantitative analysis indicated those who were in the ministry the shortest time had significantly lower secondary traumatic stress scores. This was unexpected given increased years of professional experience have been associated with decreased potential for impact (Pearlman & Mac Ian, 1995; Avary & Uhleman, 1996; Ghahramanlou & Brodbeck, 2000; Baird & Jenkins,

2003; Cunningham, 2003). Once again this finding suggested the clergy experience of secondary trauma might be less conventional than other professions. Qualitative interviews expanded on this theme and saw the emergence of a complex web of factors that appear to make longer service more of a risk for clergy than a protective factor.

Compounding issues previously discussed such as knowing the primary victims before the trauma happened, being involved at the actual scene of the trauma, the on-going relationships or exposure to these individuals once the trauma has passed were all described by participants. Also, the issue of availability of access and the demands of being expected to manage a diverse range of issues were seen as salient for many clergy. The combination of these factors provides an environment not normally seen with other professions historically associated with secondary trauma. Professions such as counsellors, mental health professionals, medical staff and first responders tend to be exposed to traumatised individuals either at the point of crisis or in the period following. Furthermore, they normally see these individuals within their workplace and not their home. Also, these professions tend to have clear professional boundaries put in place such as surgery/office hours, being off duty and the understanding that clients will not have access to them on a 24/7 basis, in an attempt to offer some sort of protection for the professional.

Clergy experiencing problems in maintaining clear personal boundaries have emerged before within the literature although the issue of trauma work was not the focus of these studies (Hill et al., 2003; Crisp-Han et al., 2011). Given the complexities of demarcation between personal and professional elements of the role have been raised before, it is hardly surprising to see them transfer into this element of the ministry. When these elements are considered, one begins to understand how those they care for are often able to permeate all aspects of their lives, potentially allowing trauma to infiltrate not only their professional but their personal domain. Therefore, the longer the cleric is in their role the more binding these complexities appear to be and as such those who are in the same parish over a sustained period of time appear to increase their risk of secondary impact.

Pfeil (2006) published a discussion article related to the impact upon clergy who provide training for the avoidance of sexual misconduct. This reflective piece based upon professional and personal experiences places emphasis on the need for clergy to recognise that in providing care for others they need to embed care for themselves. It was interesting to examine the author's personal recollections of the impact her work as a facilitator for training to avoid sexual misconduct has had upon her. She addresses issues that appear to be encouraged within ministerial life such as over functioning which led her to question the '*complex expectations*' placed upon clergy and suggests that compassion fatigue may emerge in the chasm between the expectations placed upon the cleric by their congregation and the realities of their clergy role.

She offers a humorous example of what she argues is 'coded language' in relation to an advertisement for a pastor. The advert read as follows. '*Solo pastor, joyful in the Lord, wanted by rural church. Preaching must have passion and humour. Our shepherd will also be compassionate in providing needed pastoral* care'. Pfeil (2006) suggests a more realistic translation should read. '*Self-reliant pastor, never moody, wanted by isolated church. Preaching must entertain, sooth, not challenge us. Like Jesus, our self-emptying shepherd will be available in every crisis*'. She goes on to advocate the importance of seminary colleges in providing adequate preparation for the realistic demands of ministry, including recognising their vulnerability and addressing the personal and professional costs this work may demand and the value of clergy actively seeking supportive environments that allow them to reflect on these costs.

This chapter has explored in detail the small number of studies that have focused specifically on the impact upon clergy when involved in trauma work. The exploration clearly indicated clergy are indirectly involved in trauma on many fronts ranging from major trauma events to those individual heart breaking life experiences encountered by much of humanity. For many this involvement carries personal and professional costs.

Given the picture that is painted within this chapter it is necessary to understand how these individuals are being supported and cared for when, for them, caring begins to hurt. Therefore, the following chapter will explore what is revealed within the literature about training and support in this area for clergy.

Chapter 6

I'm Holding you but Who is Holding me? Training & Support in the Ministry

The previous chapter explored how clergy are exposed to trauma and crisis and the ways in which many appear to be bearing the cost from these encounters. This naturally leads on to a consideration of the various ways in which clergy may be supported for this specific element of their pastoral role. Observations and insights of other professions who are vicariously exposed to trauma are also examined in order to build a fuller picture of what appears necessary to be in place for this work. These are all essential elements that require consideration not only to help individual clerics but also to help guide those with responsibility for clergy training and preparation for the ministry.

Support for clergy when dealing with trauma is essential as the secondary traumatisation literature clearly identifies that professional caregivers need assistance with resolving the effects of helping others through traumatic experiences (Figley, 1995, 2002a; Pearlman & Saakvitne, 1995a, 1995b, 1995c; Gentry, 2002).

Hendron (2013) offers valuable insights to a range of factors associated with training and support for crisis work within the ministry. Whilst a caveat must be put in place here as her results only examined clergy within one of the four main churches in Ireland, they are still valuable as they offer a glimpse into one of the largest sectors of clergy within the island of Ireland. Within a sample of 226 clergy, 188 reported that neither their initial theological training nor subsequent training had included working with trauma. Indeed, many clerics who did report some element of trauma training stated that it was often too brief, inadequate or undertaken as a 'box ticking' exercise. Deficiencies in training appear to have resulted in many feeling inadequately prepared for what they were faced with once they were out in their pastoral ministry. They also felt ill equipped to recognise or mange the personal impact of this work.

Clergy perceptions of their awareness and preparation for the impact of this work through their training were also explored. Very few agreed that their initial or subsequent training had made them aware of the risk of impact or prepared them for this impact should it occur. This is a worrying insight given that Stamm (2002) advocates the importance of educating care-givers regarding the potential for their work to become either harmful or life changing in an attempt to reduce secondary trauma. Training in being prepared for trauma work has been identified as a protective factor against increased levels of impact. Gentry et al. (2004) in a study examining the effectiveness of Certified Compassion Fatigue Specialist Training amongst 83 mental health professionals reported a statistically significant decrease in participants' compassion fatigue and burnout symptoms and increases in compassion satisfaction amongst those who had undergone this training scheme. Chrestman (1995) found additional training decreased the PTSD symptoms in counsellors working with trauma. Ortlepp & Friedman (2002) reported specialised training served as a protective factor amongst lay trauma counsellors.

The importance of training appears to be echoed by the voices of those who carry out the work. In their study Follette at al. (1994) reported 96% of mental health professionals said education was crucial for them to be able to cope effectively with their sexual abuse clients. Although Holaday et al. (2001) did not examine pastors' levels of training, qualitative questions relating to what advice would serving clergy give new pastors revealed 'gaining adequate training and support before working with parishioners' as the most frequently offered advice. Pearlman & Saakvitne (1995a) strongly advocate agencies employing professionals have a responsibility to help their employees to decrease the effects of the work and training is one way this can be achieved.

Poor preparation of the clergy for elements of their role is not restricted to one study or the topic of secondary impact but is reflective of studies across a range of clergy populations. Beaumont (2011) examined counselling as an element of the pastoral role amongst a sample of 758 Australian clergy and reported 46.47% received no formal counselling training. In a similar vein O'Kane and Millar (2001) investigated the counselling type work of Roman Catholic priests in Northern Ireland. Part of their questionnaire asked priests to comment on the theological and practical elements of their training. In relation to the practical element, 70% of priests rated it as largely irrelevant.

Given adequate preparation is highlighted within the literature as a prerequisite for reducing the risk of secondary trauma, clergy may potentially be placed at additional risk due to lack of adequate preparation. Many clerics may feel ill equipped for the demands and challenges of 21st century ministry because their training has neither provided them with the necessary skills and knowledge to undertake this work nor prepared them for the potential impact from it. Those responsible for clergy training need to ensure they are adequately preparing individuals for the work ahead.

Whilst clergy are not mental health professionals or counsellors, they are clearly encountering many of the experiences normally seen within the therapeutic process and as such they need some level of competence not only to recognise and seek appropriate assistance but also to have the knowledge and tools to help them recognise and manage the manifestations of any impact.

Focus now turns to how clergy might cope with the fallout from involvement in crisis work. Holaday et al. (2001) identified clergy coping strategies as '*very creative*'. These included prayer as a main factor; taking active steps to protect family time; setting workable boundaries on their work schedule; refraining from bringing too much emotional burden home to spouses and families; having a wide circle of social support; emotional distancing from what they hear; undertaking sports and hobbies; having access to staff trained in counselling; and the benefits of having additional forms of employment. The authors also raised the issue of the lack of support in the form of supervision for clergy who are experiencing secondary impact. The use of a support network has been hailed as a factor that helps to manage any negative impacts (Pearlman, 1995; Figley, 1999). In relation to these participants, the authors commented that whilst encountering similar material to mental health professionals, these clergy did not have access to supervision or structured organisational support. It was also noted that one who had been involved in peer group support indicated there was often a reticence amongst clergy to reveal they were experiencing any impact as this could be construed by their peers as incompetence and personal vulnerability.

Galek et al. (2011) also examined the variable of 'social support' as a moderator for coping with secondary traumatic stress and burnout. Social support was broken into two components emanating from within organisational structures such as supervisors and peers, and support from personal structures such as family and friends. Secondary traumatic stress was inversely related to personal support but was not significantly related to organisational support. The authors hypothesised this may be due to the fact that chaplains work in isolation within a health setting and may have limited access to their peers and supervisors. Additionally, they suggest there is a lack of congruence amongst other health professionals as to the role of chaplains within hospitals, therefore chaplains may also have limited support from their non-cleric co-workers.

In measuring social support Galek et al. (2011) used four adapted items from Frese (1999). These items explore how participants perceive, on a 4-point scale, their personal and organisational networks willingness to listen to them talk about work related issues etc. Therefore, it could be argued that whilst offering valuable insights into participant's perceptions of support, they did not actually investigate what form organisational support took (i.e., was supervision a compulsory part of their role?) and the non-association between secondary traumatic stress and organisational support may reflect the quality of support or how easily it is accessed.

Levy et al. (2011) examined how U.S. Air Force chaplains responded to working in warzones. Employing the use of the term 'compassion fatigue' to capture negative impact results indicated these chaplains did not endorse high levels of such impact but instead experienced positive psychological growth from their encounters. Regression analysis showed counselling stress exposure had a dual effect in that it predicted negative impact and posttraumatic growth.

Hendron (2013) reported poor organisational support available in terms of provision of formal supervision structures and when support was available it was often a disjointed approach. Some Diocese offered voluntary support, accessed at clergy request, whilst others appear to have no formal support in place. Exploring this subject qualitatively uncovered that for some, the absence of organisational support appears to be intrinsically linked with deep feelings of abandonment and isolation. Feelings such as these may have further knock-on effects, eating away at any sense of satisfaction the individual might gain from their work which in turn may further increase any negative feelings they have about this work.

There were also clear indications that others such as spouses and peers were being accessed on an informal basis, potentially driven by the lack of formal structures, and this appeared to be having a third level impact on some of these individuals. Clergy using their families as support structures is not a new thing. McMinn et al. (2005) reported clergy rely mainly on family members as a coping mechanism. However, this reliance can lead to pressure on family members and pressures faced by clergy can impact their marriages. Murphy-Geiss (2011) states that hiring a protestant minister is often viewed as a '*two for one deal*' and that spouses' contributions to the ministry as '*not formally acknowledged, but widely expected*'.

Within the secondary trauma literature, family members have been identified as a vital resource. Harrison & Westwood's (2009) study identifying protective factors against vicarious trauma amongst mental health therapists listed family as being valuable in providing separation and balance between professional and personal life. Paramedics in the Regehr et al. (2002) study identified the importance of home '*where they could be safe from the stressors of* work'. When such comments are contrasted with the clergy scenario where spouses are pseudo members of the ministry, it becomes clear there is little hope of separation or balance between the cleric's personal and professional life as their spouse is strongly involved in both domains.

Peers are also accessed as a means of support and this may initially be viewed as a positive strategy. Pearlman & Mac Ian (1993) found 85% of their sample of trauma counsellors used peers as the most common method for dealing with the effects of vicarious trauma. Additionally, peers are seen as serving as an important resource in managing secondary trauma (Catherall, 1995; Dyregrov & Mitchell; 1996; Saakvitne & Pearlman, 1996; Phelps et al., 2009). However, given the concerns raised previously regarding passing on impact through listening to other clergy, the instance of peers being accessed may not always be a positive thing.

Hendron (2013) highlighted that many clergy perceive their superiors and parishioners to be unsympathetic regarding their need of support and this in turn had the detrimental effect of them being reticent to seek support when it was needed.

Given that formal supervision is often viewed by professions, for example in counselling, as a vital component in supporting those who work with trauma, it was interesting to note that many clergy either do not have the same understanding of supervision, or accept supervision as an integral and necessary part of this work. Instead, they often appeared to be suspicious of the term and the potentially negative professional consequences accessing it may bring.

The issue of clergy accessing supervision has been addressed within other studies. O'Kane & Millar (2001) found 47% of their sample of Catholic Priests reported accessing a professional supervisor or counsellor as a means of support for their counselling work. Whilst these authors did not explore what form this supervision took, they did suggest a lack of training in counselling could mean priests may potentially not have the necessary knowledge to use supervision effectively.

Leach & Patterson (2010) define pastoral supervision as a process wherein designated individuals come together to consider the ministry of one of the participants in an intentional and disciplined way. During this process the supervisor will watch over, evaluate and guide the supervisee in their relationships with those they care for. When such a definition is placed within the context of the current discussion then it is argued that what is taking place for many of these clergy is neither formal nor compulsory supervision, but a series of ad hoc meetings between individuals, neither of whom may be adequately trained or supported for their own crisis work, let alone helping others to deal with theirs. Additionally, it indicated many clergy do not fully understand the aim of supervision and as such remain suspicious of the concept. There are also issues around 'who' provides support, as they clearly need to be capable of recognising and embracing the value and importance of participants' faith within their work.

Given support is hailed as a factor that helps diminish the potential for disruption and distress (Dekel et al., 2006), this lack of availability and access is a concern. Pearlman & Mac Ian (1995) examining the work of trauma therapists reported therapists who did not receive supervision experienced higher levels of distress than their counterparts who received supervision. Additionally, Walker (2004), examining the supervision practices of those working with survivors of childhood abuse, proposed supervision acted as a protective factor by ensuring early recognition of and response to the impact of such work and thus protected the professional against eventual burnout and damage.

Flannely et al. (2005) reported compassion fatigue was higher amongst clergy responders to 9/11 who did not work in association with organisations such as the American Red Cross. These authors suggested it might be the training and support that such an association offers which helps to reduce the adverse effects of working with this crisis.

This discussion in relation to support raises implications for organisational practice and further research. For researchers, issues such as support need deeper qualification and should not be measured purely in terms of quantity, as this may be misleading. For example, quantitative interpretations may suggest the number of hours in supervision is insufficient to alleviate the experience when it may be the quality of the supervision that is questionable. These findings also raise organisational implications as they direct attention towards potentially inadequate support structures for clergy.

There appears to be a need for continuity across the organisation with all clergy having access to support from a source that recognises and respects the work of the ministry. McCaffrey (2004) strongly advocates practicing in the area of trauma without good support structures is ethically unsound. In relation to their formal support structures, multiple warning signs indicate clergy may be at risk. A lack of knowledge and understanding exists around supervision and what it entails, and poor recognition of its value as a means of support. This has resulted in many clergy perceiving something as a casual discussion between friends as supervision.

Hendron (2013) suggested there was some transmission of information about what was happening at the 'coal face' to those with responsibility for clergy welfare. Over a third of participants stated they discussed this aspect of their work on some level of frequency with a superior, although additional comments suggested this finding should be viewed with caution as participants indicated the 'superior' would normally be an older or more experienced cleric, (frequently those who have been their Rector during curacy). Additionally, letting those in charge know the full extent of the situation was often associated with the risk of stigma or even 'professional suicide'.

Pearlman & McKay (2008) propose that organisations which do not have open communications and effective management, especially regarding the emotional toll of one's work, may potentially be increasing their employees' risk of developing secondary trauma. When clergy studies are considered then those in charge of providing formal training and support do not appear to be stepping up to the mark either in acknowledging the difficulties of the role or making themselves available to those under their care. Given Pearlman & Saakvitne's (1995b) call that those in charge of the welfare of individuals who undertake work with trauma carry a weighty responsibility, it may be this responsibility is not being adequately met.

Understanding the reasons why clergy do not seek help would appear to be important if ways of improving this situation are to be found. Given, this is not an element of secondary trauma normally seen within the literature, Hendron's (2013) findings are valuable from both a research and practice standpoint as they provide a glimpse into the minds of individuals and their rationale for not seeking help. The web of interrelated factors involved here included organisational fear, stigma, judgement and mistrust. The issue of those in charge, or parishioners, being unsympathetic to a cleric who admitted an impact from their work and sought help was evident. Furthermore, it was clear clergy believed if they raised such an issue they would be stigmatised with a 'black mark' set against them. This mark would remain throughout their careers and would go against them when seeking advancement within their career.

The term stigma originated from the Greeks who used it when referring to bodily signs indicating there was something unusual or bad about their bearer. Goffman (1963) argues the term is employed in a similar sense in the present day but is used to represent disgrace rather than a visual bodily sign. Therefore, the negative association between asking for help and having done something wrong is extremely worrying as few individuals will seek help if they perceive what they are doing is wrong. This is not the first occurrence of clergy fearing negative reprisals if they seek support. Examining more general work related stress amongst American protestant clergy, Meek et al. (2003) identified negative reprisal as an obstacle to clergy remaining healthy. It appears the stigma of being perceived as weak, professionally incompetent, or even worse as 'spiritually bankrupt' because God is not enough to solve their problems, are factors too great to overcome in several domains of clergy work.

Killian (2008) asserts that an individual's perception of how supportive their organisation will be should they require assistance, greatly impacts their ability to manage secondary impact. Therefore, there may be fundamental issues amongst church cultures regarding their organisational ethos around acceptance and acknowledgement of impact as a natural consequence of this work.

In relation to clergy help seeking, gender also appears to be a factor that stops females from either indicating all is not well or seeking support. Hendron (2013) reported a definite sense that as a female it was more difficult to admit problems, as females are still highly aware some dissention remains regarding their ordination. They perceived that many people still think females should not be rectors and so when problems arise they do not admit to them for fear of adding fuel to the argument they are unsuited for ministry. The issue of females gaining equal status in the ministry has raised its head previously in other domains. Rayburn et al. (1986) reported females themselves and others perceived they were being unfairly treated in seminary college and in relation to selection and promotion for jobs. They also reported they were viewed with more suspicion by colleagues and congregations. These authors suggested this results in females perceiving a greater need to do better than their male counterparts.

Amongst many other professions associated with secondary impact such as mental health, nursing etc., the gender balance swings the other way and these roles are often dominated by females. It would be valuable in future to explore if amongst these professions, the issue of gender raises its head in the opposite direction with males not seeking help due to the perception that as men they should be able to cope. There were hints of this amongst male paramedics in Regehr et al.'s (2002) study where participants spoke of the "*macho atmosphere*" that deterred them from being really opened about how they were feeling. Combining this suggestion with Hendron (2013) findings points towards the perception of gender stereotypes being a barrier to the help seeking process.

Surprisingly Hendron (2013) found concerns around confidentiality and honesty. Despite high numbers discussing the impact of their work with their peers, many expressed a mistrust of sharing honestly how they felt with their peers for fear of their unburdening being shared with others or superiors and being construed as a weakness. Meek et al. (2003) examining clergy stress also found issues around who would have access to their information should they seek help, suggesting they may resist seeking help when issues of trust and confidentiality were not guaranteed. Turton (2010) reported 52% of his participants rated not being confidential as the reason they did not access a pastoral support scheme.

Given that the media has such a huge influence within society, does their view of the clergy have any influence on support seeking? Hendron (2013) found that the influence of the media emerged as a theme for not seeking help. It appears the public scrutiny of what clergy do and how they are impacted, is not viewed as a positive thing by many participants. Accounts emerged of instances where local media had not been sympathetic to clergy who experienced problems. Some participants indicated this in part has been a result of recent scandals involving Catholic clergy, especially in Ireland, which have received a high media profile and appear to have resulted in clergy even amongst other denominations feeling they cannot be perceived as being anything other than perfect in order to avoid media criticism. Quinley (1974) suggested clergy, due to the very nature of their role, are more likely than their parishioners to be attuned to what the media is presenting. However, these authors were reviewing the relationship between clergy and the media as a positive one where clergy are the holders of power. The current findings suggest clergy perceive this balance may have shifted and clergy now perceive power to be in favour of the media.

A number of additional factors appear to be salient for clergy not seeking support. The clergy role is somewhat unique in that one's home is tied up with the job and Hendron (2013) found that this was a salient issue when it comes to seeking help. The fact that if a cleric exits their role they will also be made homeless, results in some sitting on a problem rather than seeking assistance. Also salient are factors such as pensions that do not cover psychological illness. Once again this is a factor that has not been explored widely within the literature.

Although whilst not specifically addressing the concept of poor job benefits as barriers to help seeking, Pearlman & Saakvitne (1995a) suggested provision of employee benefits could decrease secondary impact. Chrestman (1995) reported evidence that increased income was related to decreased symptoms of psychological distress. There may be a lesson to learn here for those responsible for clergy welfare and those with organisational responsibility. They should strive to ensure the organisational culture is one that acknowledges, accepts and is compassionate towards the aftermath of this work. This concern and compassion could be communicated through ensuring pension and insurance provision are adequate should the impact become too much and individuals require additional assistance.

This chapter has highlighted that this crucial aspect of the clergy role has often lacked adequate preparation, training and support. The lack of these key elements places clerics at an enhanced risk of vicarious impact and as such should be a major concern not only for individual clerics but for those who hold organisation and parish responsibility for their care and wellbeing.

Chapter 7

And now for the Good News: Compassion Satisfaction & Joy in the Pastoral Ministry

Herman (1992) proposed that working with trauma can have its rewards as well as costs, going on to suggest that the work may even be enriching for the professional undertaking it through increasing their appreciation for life and facilitating deeper insights into themselves. Therefore, it seemed appropriate if indeed a little counterintuitive, to bring this book towards a conclusion with a chapter that highlights some of the positive aspects of working with crisis and goes on to explore one of the positive strategies for recognising and managing the negative cost of caring.

Given the discussion of the previous chapters it may be hard to imagine that a positive side to this work even exists, however a positive side to trauma work is now both recognised and accepted and therefore it is possible that for some working with trauma in the Pastoral Ministry it may also evoke a positive response. Given that authors such as Case et al. (2020) contend that clergy provide significant support to their congregations and at times this comes at a cost to their mental wellbeing, this chapter advocates the salient need to identify any factors that might enable clergy to flourish in the face of these occupational stressors. This understanding is also essential to ensure that any prevention and intervention efforts designed to support clergy and their well-being are accurately informed and specifically targeted to their unique needs. As such this chapter will briefly examine conversations around positive elements to trauma work before exploring in detail the potential benefits of the concept of emotional intelligence as a salient factor in being able to recognize and manage any impact from involvement in trauma work.

So how does such emotionally demanding and challenging work result in something that is enriching and affirmative? The work of Beth Stamm which has been discussed within previous chapters in relation to the negative impact of trauma work is an excellent starting point. Stamm (2002) postulates that a positive aspect to this work does exist and as such she attempted to capture it with the term compassion satisfaction. This, she suggested is related to the satisfaction individuals derive from being able to carry out their role well. It can involve feeling optimistic about being able to contribute positively to society as well as deriving enjoyment from being able to offer help to those in need.

The evolving mind-set, that there could be joy as well as sorrow derived from trauma work led Radey & Figley (2007) to argue that there needs to be a shift in the paradigm in which this emotionally challenging work is viewed and instead of focusing solely on avoidance of the negative, focus should also be directed towards the positive fulfilment the work can also bring. Ludick & Figley (2017) added to the conversation with the introduction of the concept of compassion fatigue resilience through which there is an interplay of decreased levels of compassion fatigue and enhanced levels of resilience.

Despite the emergence of a more positive view of this challenging work few studies have directly explored it as a concept (Jacobson, 2006) and Craig & Sprang (2010) point out that whilst this topic appears to be recognised by and of interest to researchers, as a proven outcome it appears to have been excluded from much of the research. Work that has been undertaken has been sparse and results variable, suggesting that the interplay of the negative and positive may not be a straightforward process and many personal and external variables can influence the outcome for individuals.

Firstly, in relation to the negative side of the experience eroding the positive, Collins & Long (2003) offered key insights into the inverse relationship between the positive and negative impact from trauma work. Undertaking a longitudinal study, they examined the impact upon caregivers when working with acutely traumatised individuals. Data was gathered from members of multidisciplinary trauma and recovery teams who worked with survivors of the Omagh bombing in Northern Ireland in 1998. Results indicated that as levels of negative impact rose over time, levels of positive impact measured as compassion satisfaction decreased. The authors suggested that increasing demands and the detrimental impact of the work had an eroding effect on feeling any positivity from their involvement. Hooper et al. (2010) examined the variables of compassion satisfaction, compassion fatigue and burnout in emergency nurses compared to non-emergency nurses. They reported low levels of compassion satisfaction and high levels of compassion fatigue amongst all participants with emergency nurses reporting lower levels of compassion satisfaction than staff in other specialties. However, these authors found only a weak association between compassion satisfaction and compassion fatigue.

Conrad & Kellar-Guenther (2006) examined the positive and negative impact of their work upon 363 child protection workers in Colorado. They reported an inverse relationship between compassion satisfaction and both compassion fatigue and burnout. We must recognise that other factors may also be at play here and correlation does not prove causation. However, this does suggest that as levels of satisfaction increase, levels of more negative impact decrease, therefore, this satisfaction is potentially a mitigating factor for negative impact.

Yet other studies have shown that involvement in trauma work can result in a positive response. In an earlier study, Steed & Dowling (1998) whilst not specifically addressing the concept of growth, found their respondents reported an increased appreciation of life and personal growth when involved in trauma work. Examining family violence workers, Bell (2003) discovered 40% of participants, felt they had become more grateful for life and less judgmental of others. Building on such proposals Arnold et al. (2005) presented the associated concept of vicarious posttraumatic growth, reporting that therapists noticed changes in themselves, their perspectives of life and their evaluations of the forces driving human nature. Adding further flesh to these bones Robins et al. (2009) explored compassion fatigue, compassion satisfaction and burnout amongst 314 health care providers in a children's hospital. Their study employed multiple regression techniques to produce a model of factors influencing levels of compassion fatigue. Results indicated higher compassion satisfaction was associated with non-trainee status, using external coping strategies, greater cognitive/affective empathy, and lower blurring of caregiver boundaries.

Naturally, the positive side of the trauma experience for clergy is relevant to this chapter. As previously mentioned, Stamm (2002) attempted to capture the positive side of trauma work and this was done within the ProQOL Scale via the compassion satisfaction subscale. Using this measurement scale Hendron (2013) found that 25.2% of her clergy participants reported high levels of compassion satisfaction. Whilst this percentage was almost identical to that suggested by the scale's normative data for other professions, the fact that only around a quarter of clergy participants indicated these higher levels did appear to somewhat go against the grain of prior research and suggestions that clergy gain immense satisfaction from their role (Fletcher, 1990; Grosh & Olsen, 2000; Crossley, 2002).

At this juncture, it is worth recognising that even the concept of satisfaction with their role is a complex one for clergy and one that researchers and authors have found difficult to definitively capture. For example, clergy satisfaction has by some been discussed in terms of their unwillingness to endorse what could be perceived as the secular definition of satisfaction. Turton (2010) contended some clergy resent their role being defined as just a 'job' when they see it as a sacred calling. Consequently, the idea that a 'calling' could be assessed in terms of satisfaction and dissatisfaction as with secular roles is difficult for many to admit or relate to. Clergy at times seem to battle between attending to their personal needs versus their professional obligation to attend to the needs of others.

In a similar vein Francis et al. (2011) suggest religious leaders are often reluctant to endorse concepts associated with self-seeking pleasure, gratification and indulgence and therefore clergy may be unwilling to commit to paper any indication of self-satisfaction as an important element of their role.

This portraying a positive public image of ministry is articulated by Abernethy (2002) who, in a painfully honest account of the personal challenges and costs of his ministry states, *"There is a danger we portray the glittering image and not our real humanity"* (p51). This appears to support the thoughts of Rayburn et al. (1986) who contended that social desirability is a factor that prevents many clergy from admitting to many of the strains associated with their role.

Due to the very nature of their vocation or calling, clergy may feel it is expected they should portray a high sense of fulfilment through serving God and helping others. Hendron (2013) noted this 'keeping up appearances' during qualitative interviews as many clergy who scored highly in relation to negative impact appeared on first meeting to be relatively unaffected. It was only as the interviews progressed and trust was established that stories of personal and professional struggles emerged. Clergy did admit to gaining satisfaction from different elements of their role such as preaching and bible teaching from which they drew great joy.

However, trauma involvement was one aspect many reported finding challenging and one for which they felt ill prepared and poorly supported.

Naturally, having any additional personal tools that can assist an individual to more positively manage any negative impact is an area that requires attention. Hendron (2013) offered valuable insights here with a factor that should be of personal and organisational interest to those who work with trauma. Her study exploring the experience of clergy working with trauma within the pastoral ministry had the additional element of examining the influence of the concept of emotional intelligence (Mayer & Salovey, 1997) within this clergy experience. The concept of emotional intelligence is shown as a personal factor that may potentially assist with recognition and management of negative impact upon clergy from their involvement within trauma work, however, Hendron et al (2012) contended that despite the growing diversity of concepts and occupations that emotional intelligence has been associated with, those within religious domains appear to have slipped under the radar of researchers.

Morrison's (2007) proposal that emotional intelligence is not an end in itself but instead should be viewed as a way in which to enrich thinking and action, is particularly salient for the discussion of this chapter as the following discussion will suggest that it may be advantageous in increasing positive impact and thus indirectly decreasing negative impact and as such could be a valuable tool in increasing resilience. Therefore, Hendron's (2013) exploration of emotional intelligence as a factor that may potentially enable individuals to recognise impact, understand the cause of impact and seek adaptive coping strategies to help manage the impact was highly valuable not only to clergy and the Pastoral Ministry but also beyond, to other professionals involved in the care and support of others.

Hendron's (2013) initial assumption that emotional intelligence could be of value within the experience of working with trauma within the Pastoral Ministry was based upon the theoretical construct of emotional intelligence and several related studies. Firstly, Mayer & Salovey (1997) suggested that those with higher levels of emotional intelligence pay attention to and understand their emotional data, making them more able to:

- Identify emotion in their physical states, feelings and thoughts and to express these emotions accurately,

- Use emotional data to facilitate their thinking to generate judgements and encourage specific approaches to problems,

- Have the ability to understand complex emotions that result from the blending and transition of emotional data and

- Have the ability to reflectively engage with or detach themselves from emotions and to manage emotions in themselves by moderating negative emotions or enhancing pleasant ones.

Salovey & Mayer (1990) had already suggested links between higher emotional intelligence and improved psychological wellbeing and furthermore emotional intelligence had been identified within a number of studies as a dynamic that could intercede between stress and health (Salovey et al., 2002; Slaski & Cartwright, 2002; Extremera & Fernández-Berrocal, 2005). Also the influence of emotional intelligence within wider concepts such as role satisfaction (Wong & Law, 2002; Sy et al., 2006; Kafetsios & Zampetakis, 2008); and also emotional intelligence and the processes of coping (Pau & Croucher, 2003; Riley & Schutte, 2003).

Hendron (2013) proposed the role of emotional intelligence within the wider workplace also merited recognition as Matthews et al. (2004, p470) argue, "*Work related emotional intelligence competencies are vital if one is to successfully negotiate the demands, constraints, and opportunities necessary to succeed in the workplace*". Matthews and his colleagues further suggested emotional intelligence might be linked to several aspects of occupational life that were of particular interest (i.e., satisfaction and coping with occupational stress).

Whilst much of the existing emotional intelligence literature had focused on the organisational and retail domains, interest in the potential value of emotional intelligence is beginning to seep into the more 'caring professions'. For example, studies have emerged suggesting the importance of emotional intelligence amongst: medical students (Austin et al., 2007); nurses (Akerjordet & Severinsson, 2004, 2007, 2009; Gooch, 2006) and Morrison (2007) discussed the potential value of it within social work. Additionally, associations have also been reported between emotional intelligence and the impact of primary trauma (Hunt & Evans, 2004).

Matthews et al. (2004) reported links between emotional intelligence and coping with occupational stress whilst Jordan et al. (2002) propose the concept assists individuals to employ better coping strategies when dealing with work. Bates (2005) examined the role of emotional, cognitive and social factors upon secondary traumatic stress amongst a sample of human service professionals. Whilst results reported no significant relationship between total emotional intelligence and the subscales of secondary traumatic stress or compassion satisfaction, they did find a significant negative correlation between the experiential emotional intelligence and secondary traumatic stress and a positive correlation between the emotional intelligence branch of managing emotions and compassion satisfaction. Compassion satisfaction was also positively associated with the emotional intelligence task scores for sensations and emotional relations.

This led Bates (2005) to suggest those with reduced abilities to perceive emotions and those who have difficulty in expressing how they are feeling and comparing these feelings with other sensory experiences, may be at greater risk of experiencing secondary traumatic stress and highlights the importance of emotional abilities in coping with secondary impact. She also suggested a sense of achievement was linked to the ability to appropriately experience emotions and to use these experiences appropriately within future decision-making. The opposite of this behaviour would be the suppression or ignoring of emotions in decision-making that could result in less satisfaction in one's role.

In examining emotional intelligence specifically related to clergy and trauma work within the pastoral ministry, Hendron (2013) revealed negative moderate associations between the subscales of emotional intelligence and secondary traumatic stress and emotional intelligence and burnout. She also found a strong positive correlation between emotional intelligence and compassion satisfaction. These were valuable results as they suggested interactions between emotional intelligence and several recognised aspects of the experience of working vicariously with trauma.

Morrison (2007) highlighted the significance of this conceptualisation of emotional intelligence in placing emotions alongside thinking and action. This resonated with the view of Hendron's presentation of emotional intelligence not as an end in itself but as a means to enrich thinking, action and outcomes, all of which are vital components in counteracting secondary impact.

In a less related but still important comparison study, Kwako et al. (2011) tried to determine if emotional intelligence and social support differed between patients who had a major depressive disorder (MDD) and healthy individuals. Results indicated that those with MDD had lower emotional intelligence and lower levels of social support. The study's authors suggested the ability to use emotional data and to act appropriately upon it may be beneficial in the management of MDD. In the main, association between emotional intelligence and our abilities to recognise, use, understand and manage our emotional data have been examined through a quantitative lens.

However, McLaughlin (2008) advocates interest in and relevance of a theory really becomes alive when links are made between it and lived experiences. Hendron's (2013) study stepped beyond the quantitative realm of measuring emotional intelligence levels and its associations and shifted the paradigm into the qualitative. This movement beyond the quantitative validation of emotional intelligence has been identified as rare yet necessary (Smollan & Parry, 2011) and therefore places Hendon's findings in a unique position of providing a dual understanding of emotional intelligence with the secondary traumatisation experience. The study's ethos of seeking clarification and deeper understanding through viewing principles not only through statistical analysis but through actual experiences builds upon Funder's (2001) arguments that concepts such as emotional intelligence should be understood in terms of their 'real world' behaviours.

The picture that emerged was one of emotional intelligence certainly not offering guaranteed protection against secondary impact. In fact, higher levels may potentially put some individuals at risk through their propensity to empathise and become overly involved emotionally with parishioners' issues. However, enhanced levels of emotional intelligence did appear to facilitate self-monitoring for and recognition of impact and to facilitate more positive management strategies such as seeking suitable interpersonal support in the form of supervision or medical assistance. It also may act as a buffer against developing severe cognitive disruptions through the undertaking of active recognition and coping strategies and through enhancing a more positive view of the work and thus increasing satisfaction gleaned from it.

The combination of these influences may result in those with higher emotional intelligence being less likely to exit their ministry early. There were clear themes pertaining to emotional intelligence within the experience of working with trauma. Distinct differences were noted between participants' emotional intelligence in relation to recognising the impact from this work. Some with lower levels of emotional intelligence chose to speak of the impact in others rather than themselves and it was difficult to gauge if these individuals were willing or unable to connect how they felt with trauma work. In contrast those with higher levels of emotional intelligence appeared to adopt a completely different approach and spoke of how they monitor and detect signs within themselves that all is not well. This often involved a conscious process of watching out for telltale signs emerging from physical, emotional or behavioural symptoms which they appeared to be able to connect as resulting from incidents within their pastoral visits or to being involved in a long-term cycle of providing emotional support for others.

This is an extremely important strategy that emotional intelligence can potentially enhance, given that early detection of secondary impact through self-monitoring and awareness is identified as a key preventative to developing severe distress (Oswald, 1991; Phelps et al., 2009). It is also salient in light of Pearlman & Saakvitne's (1995b) suggestion that low self awareness places an individual at risk of secondary impact and also that recognition and engagement with one's emotional reaction to any stressor is necessary in order for the stressor to be cognitively integrated (Lepore et al., 2000).

Emotional intelligence involves the ability to perceive and accurately express emotion (Mayer & Salovey, 1997) and the dimension of recognising and expressing emotions is present in virtually every emotional intelligence instrument (Ciarrochi & Scott, 2006). The ability to recognise emotional data is hailed as a positive skill contributing to wellbeing, whilst on the other hand, difficulty in recognising and expressing emotions, has been related to decreased wellbeing and depression (Ciarrochi et al., 2002) and somatisation in patients (Bach & Bach, 1995). Additionally, the ability to recognise and express feelings is associated with better psychological adjustment (Lepore & Smyth, 2002).

There have long been associated benefits of attending to and working through one's emotions in relation to traumatic experiences (Horowitz, 1976). Stanton et al. (2000) hypothesise that coping through an emotional approach in breast cancer patients would enhance adjustment to their condition which could then improve their health status. Their findings reported this to be true, especially in the short to medium term when emotional focusing was beneficial. This is especially relevant for Hendron (2013) when discussing those with higher emotional intelligence who did appear to focus on their emotions with more clarity and thus potentially reduced their secondary traumatic stress levels.

Ramos et al. (2007) examined the benefits of perceived emotional intelligence facilitating cognitive and emotional processing of acute stressors and found emotional clarity worked first on a preventive level and suggested being able to discriminate between ones' emotions whilst facing stressful encounters is a beneficial initial skill in cognitive adaption. In light of Bride et al.'s (2003) counsel that self-monitoring for symptoms of secondary trauma may help in positive management of the experience emotional intelligence appears to be a positive tool. However, Stanton et al. (2000) also reported that focusing long term on the same emotional data without having any strategies to reduce these feelings resulted in greater anxiety over time. There is a fine line to be drawn between the benefits of attending to emotions and the counterproductive strategy of paying these emotions too much attention, leading to rumination.

Salovey et al. (1999) addressed this when advocating the benefits of emotional intelligence in the coping process. Rumination is defined as submissively and repeatedly focusing on one's signs of distress and the situations surrounding those signs (Nolen-Hoeksema et al., 2008). Rumination has previously been positively associated with depressed mood (Nolen-Hoeksema, 1991). In line with emotional intelligence theory, Salovey et al. (1999) present appraising and recognising emotions and the ability to articulate these emotions as the most basic of all emotional intelligence abilities. They also recognise individuals vary in relation to how much attention they pay to emotions and their mood states and purport those who pay too much attention to perceiving and appraising their emotions are more likely to indulge in ruminative behaviour. Leading them to suggest moderate attention to ones' moods may be advantageous whilst elevated levels of attention may be counterproductive to the coping process.

This is an important consideration within religious organisational settings, especially if there appears to be a less robust organisational ethos towards recognition of and support for any potential negative impact. As such, if an individual recognises they are being impacted by their work and are restricted by the organisational structure from openly addressing and seeking help for this impact then these individuals may potentially be worse off as they recognise impact but have nowhere to take it. Recognising impact is only one step in the successful journey to positive management of secondary trauma and strategies that facilitate successful adaption and assimilation of the experience are necessary progress steps (Saakvitne & Pearlman, 1996; Harrison & Westwood, 2009; Stamm, 2009).

It is also of interest to explore if individuals can use their prior emotional experiences to set in place strategies that will help protect them in similar experiences in the future. Using emotional foresight for positive outcomes has previously been highlighted. Caruso & Salovey (2004, p124) use the term "*predicting the emotional future*". Based upon the understanding that emotions have rules and following patterns, if we understand and recognise them, can potentially identify in advance how we will be affected and react to particular experiences. Dunn et al. (2007) referred to the term "*affective forecasting*" (p85). Exploring individual differences in affective forecasting they reported the ability to accurately forecast was related to emotional intelligence as measured by the MSCEIT instrument with the emotional management domain emerging as the most critical for these predictions.

Studies have also been undertaken which revealed a similar vein of thought regarding the adaptive use of emotional data. Isen (2001) reported associations between the positive affect and an enhanced ability to assess a situation. Kusche &

Greenberg (2001) drew distinctions between the development of emotional competencies through training programmes such as PATHS (Promoting Alternative Thinking Strategies) and alleviating emotional distress and enhancing social adaption. Hunt & Evans (2004), examining the influence of emotional intelligence on responses to experiences of primary trauma, found individuals with higher emotional intelligence reported fewer psychological symptoms related to their traumatic experience due in part to those with higher emotional intelligence being more likely to adopt a monitoring style of processing the trauma. This process of monitoring may well be linked to the processes involved in employing emotional foresight as a monitoring tool.

Hendron (2013) found that those with higher emotional intelligence were more likely to employ emotional foresight as a positive tool in their experiences. These individuals frequently spoke of understanding in advance how they could be negatively impacted by elements of their trauma work. This appeared frequently based on a learned experience process built on recollections of how they felt and behaved during previous experiences. Recognition that they could be affected by a situation resulted in several positive strategies being undertaken to moderate the blow.

Firstly, independent support strategies were often put in place before they were needed; some ensuring these were in place even before they entered the ministry. On other occasions advance strategies to manage difficult upcoming encounters which they knew from past experiences may be problematic, were devised. This is valuable considering Phelps et al. (2009) setting out preventative and management strategies for secondary impact. They identified risk assessments of particular aspects of their roles as having the potential to evoke a distressing response as an essential tool for the professional and directing attention towards emotional intelligence as a positive tool for facilitating the scanning and assessment of personal risk.

It is also worth comparing the picture at the other end of the emotional intelligence spectrum and the opposite of 'emotional foresight' was termed by Hendron (2013) as 'emotional blindside'. Those with lower levels of emotional intelligence did not appear to use their emotional data history as a predictor of future emotional impact and it appeared by not employing this strategy they were feeling like ships tossed at sea, unable to control events and at the mercy of the many crisis they encountered. Whilst Hendron (2013) did not wish to present an unrealistic suggestion that emotional intelligence is a crystal ball guaranteeing those who possess it prior knowledge of events and an unaffected encounter, there did clearly appear to be some value in being emotionally fore-warned and thus potentially emotionally fore-armed. Whilst this may not always prevent negative impact, it may enable them to feel more in control of events and have support in place should signs of impact emerge and as such placed emotional intelligence as a valuable tool within the secondary traumatisation experience.

Interestingly, Hendron (2013) also found that higher emotional intelligence participants favoured the use of metaphors in what appeared to be an attempt to draw others into their world and find common ground or shared reality. It may be that emotional intelligence, by providing these individuals with a more developed emotional vocabulary, helped them to more effectively share how they feel. This may motivate them to seek help more readily as they feel able to express their experiences, be understood and potentially helped.

The inability to express emotions is defined as alexithymia (Sifneos, 1972) and difficulty in expressing emotions has been identified as predicting inferior psychological adjustment (Pennebaker, 1997; Lepore & Smith, 2002). It has also been associated with signs of stress (Wassel, 2002). Emotional intelligence has previously been reported as being strongly inversely related to alexithymia (Parker et al., 2001). Trinidad et al. (2004) examined emotional intelligence as a protective strategy against smoking in adolescents and reported emotional intelligence was associated with higher perceived ability to refuse offers of cigarettes. This they suggest resulted from their emotional intelligence enabling them to understand their feelings regarding the negative impact of smoking and making them able to articulate these feelings in words. Since there has been limited examination of emotional intelligence and favouring metaphors as a means of transferring one's personal experience to the realms of another individual's understanding Hendron's (2013) findings suggest that this could be explored as an important step in developing our understanding as to how emotional intelligence manifests itself in situations such as sharing life's experiences.

Morrison (2007) frankly states a lack of emotional awareness can result in important information being missed. Addressing this issue Shulman (1990) encapsulates the importance of professionals understanding the intrapersonal and interpersonal domains of emotions. Shulman (1990) states "*The capacity to be in touch with the client's feelings is related to the worker's ability to acknowledge his/her own*" (p156). Before a worker can understand the power of emotion in the life of the client, it is necessary to discover its importance in the worker's own experience. Therefore, any lack of insight into their own emotional databank may not only impact them but may lead them not to consider the emotions of others.

Caruso & Salovey (2004) suggest the ability to determine what is going to happen to us emotionally will fail to be of any real benefit if others involved are not considered. Using emotional knowledge will enable us to see with some degree of certainty how others, as well as ourselves, will react to certain situations. Therefore, for clergy, utilising emotional knowledge may be valuable not only for setting strategies in place to assist moderating and managing secondary impact but also to safeguard interpersonal relationships with their parishioners and thus potentially enhancing their overall pastoral ministry.

Hendron (2013) reported clergy with higher emotional intelligence appeared more able to find a realistic balance between their needs and the needs of their parishioners, with accounts of being connected to the demands of their parishioners but also striving to take steps to find ways to realistically manage these demands. These participants spoke of the value of Non-Stipend Ministers (NSMs) and retired clergy as being important in being able to provide cover for parishes whilst still ensuring some personal free time.

In the quantitative element of Hendron's study there were clues that higher emotional intelligence may prompt recognising the value of external help to manage this experience as initial statistical analysis had revealed positive relationships between higher emotional intelligence and accessing independent supervision and also discussing this work with peers and superiors. Given support has been highlighted as a positive influence in the management of secondary trauma the association between emotional intelligence and increasing accessing support should be viewed as positive. Interview conversations with higher emotional intelligence participants centred around their recognition that impact from this work could occur and therefore there was a need to seek support. Indeed, many noted that to attempt this work unsupported was foolhardy and dangerous.

Interestingly, differing emotional intelligence levels appeared to influence the choice of management strategy sought. Higher emotional intelligence was frequently associated with support in the form of interpersonal interactions in terms of supervision or building a trusted relationship with someone who understood their work and in the main these relationships appeared to involve being able to talk things through. Lower emotional intelligence participants indicated they favoured solitary pursuits and spoke of choosing heavy physical work or solitary walks. This is hardly surprising given the associations between emotional intelligence and enhanced social relationships but in this case, it may be the choice of solitary pursuits offers less opportunity for the normalisation of the experience though awareness this is a consequence of their work experienced by others. As such, the lack of structured meaningful conversations around how they are feeling may fail to allow them to successfully process and integrate their experiences. Lepore et al. (2000) examined talking as a means of facilitating cognitive and emotional adaption of acute stressors and suggested talking about the stressors could facilitate adjustment to the stressor.

Hendron (2013) also reported that emotional intelligence also appeared to make a difference to the mind-set participants adopted towards this work and its impact. Her initial quantitative results had revealed a positive association between emotional intelligence and compassion satisfaction and interviews expanded on this with mind-sets towards their role, recognition and management of impact and satisfaction derived being discussed.

The relationship between emotional intelligence and personal and professional satisfaction is not a new one. Sy et al. (2006) explored associations between emotional intelligence and employees job satisfaction amongst 187 food service employees. They reported positive associations between emotional intelligence and employees job satisfaction and performance. The results supported those of Wong & Law (2002) who had reported associations between emotional intelligence and job satisfaction amongst a sample of MBA students. Matthews et al. (2004) also reported links between emotional intelligence and increased job satisfaction.

George (1995) suggests managing moods, especially positive ones, will enhance an individual's performance at work, which will naturally influence the satisfaction they gain from the work.

Hendron (2013) suggested that overall higher emotional intelligence appeared to be associated with multiple clergy personal and professional factors; those who were able to see the positive side of this work and to view themselves as more capable of undertaking it; those who had recognised that they were ill prepared and supported for this element of their role and therefore sought training and support independently of their organisation and those who monitored for any impact upon themselves. All of this in turn appeared to result in a more positive view of their role and more feelings of satisfaction derived from it.

This was not to say they were unrealistic about the work or untouched by it. On the contrary, it appeared that many were more positive in spite of what they had been through. They spoke freely about the satisfaction they gained from being involved with others who had gone through tragic experiences. This satisfaction often grew from an enhanced appreciation of the ability of others to overcome and survive tragedy. Often this was aligned with reframing the work within their 'calling', potentially shifting the balance away from any personal level of fulfilment and placing fulfilment within the higher spiritual realm.

These participants appeared to try to make sense out of what had happened and to integrate the changed reality brought about by the trauma into something they could accept and live with. This was often done through aligning the situation with God's will, which they felt would ultimately be for good, not evil. They recognised the impact of this work but would not have had it any other way, viewing the personal cost of the work as well worth being involved on a personal level with victims and survivors of trauma. Some viewed what little training they received in a more positive light, which may have resulted in them perceiving themselves as more able to undertake this work.

In contrast those at the lower end of the emotional intelligence spectrum paint a less rosy picture of their work with trauma and their ministry in general. Often at times presenting it as a negative experience and adopting a fatalistic approach that they could not avoid this negative work. This builds upon work that has previously associated higher emotional intelligence with increased self-efficacy (Azizian & Samadi, 2012) which in turn has been associated with approaching difficult tasks more confidently, (Bandura et al., 2003).

It may be those with higher emotional intelligence perceive they are more adept at dealing with the difficult tasks of caring for those who experience tragedy and this attitude towards their work and their ability to undertake it may indirectly help them to manage some of the challenges of the work through cognitive reframing which increases the satisfaction they gain from the work. Benight & Harper (2002) reported self-efficacy acted as a mediator against the onset of psychological distress amongst various traumatic events. Therefore, consideration of emotional intelligence as a factor in the process of increasing self-efficacy that potentially influences positive perceptions of the work and goes on to increase the satisfaction an individual derives from their work may merit consideration during clergy training.

More positive attitudes and comments of participants with higher emotional intelligence echo those of therapists in Harrison & Westwood's (2009) study who spoke in terms of '*active optimism*' (p210) and '*exquisite empathy*' (p213) as helping them manage the impact from their work. These authors reported that contrary to aspects being viewed only as negative factors, their participants viewed them as sustaining forces in their work. Engstrom et al. (2008) also touches on a similar thread contending the cost of empathic connection is necessary for developing vicarious resilience which Hernández et al. (2007) presented as recognising that challenging work can have a positive side. Engstrom et al. (2008) carried out a study examining vicarious resilience amongst 10 therapists working with torture victims. They suggested vicarious resilience may occur through the professional applying lessons from their clients' resilience to their own lives, which in turn allows the professional to reframe their own troubles and through this process they may be better able to cope with their personal difficulties.

McLaughlin (2008) identifies the focus of psychology and psychotherapy appears to be shifting more towards spotlighting the more positive aspects of life such as resilience and wellbeing and giving less attention to dysfunction. The role of positive affect is now being more widely accepted as a potential moderator for life's negative experiences (Ramos et al., 2007). Vaillant (2000) in his discussion of the role of adaptive mental mechanisms proposes when social support and cognitive solutions are absent, then resilience will emerge amongst mental defences which alter perceptions of external and internal realities. Vaillant's statement is important in relation to the picture painted by this study of clergy who due to the very nature of their role may have little or no escape from exposure to the difficult material of others or the ability to alter tragic situations. Therefore, in situations such as the pastoral ministry, where there are no practical solutions to the avoidance of trauma work, the value of emotional intelligence enhancing mental defences and allowing individuals to place unchangeable difficult situations in more positive mindsets certainly is a valuable finding and one which merits further exploration as a resilience tool.

This more positive mindset may also be a way in which we begin to see insights to why those with higher emotional intelligence may potentially have fewer disruptions in their cognitive schemas. The value of emotional intelligence enhancing the ability to frame events less negatively has previously been examined. Schutte et al. (2002) reported positive relationships between emotional intelligence and being able to generate and maintain a positive mood despite attempts being made to induce a negative mood. Higher scores on emotional intelligence have also been associated with positive perspective taking (Schutte et al., 2001).

Ehlers et al. (2010) investigated the effectiveness of cognitive interventions on post traumatic stress disorder and indicated they were a feasible alternative treatment. There may also be further benefits from adopting a more optimistic mindset. Gross (2002) proposed strategies which people adopt to regulate their emotions often impact their relationships. It is well recognised the expression of amiable emotions is more likely to elicit approval from others whilst the expression of negative emotions often drives others away (Argyle & Lu, 1990; Furr & Funder, 1998). Therefore, when impacted by one's involvement in trauma, the adoption of a positive outlook may have a helpful knock-on effect upon interpersonal relationships, which in turn can provide valuable support and perspective.

McCann & Pearlman (1990c) suggest it is all too easy for those who are exposed to the trauma and crisis of life to take on the mantra that life and the world are terrible places and thus increase their risk of negative impact. If those with higher levels of emotional intelligence are less likely to adopt this mantra then it may be a valuable asset when attempting to readdress the balance between the negative and positive aspects of the work.

Hendron (2013) also highlighted differences in the type of empathic connection between emotional intelligence and secondary traumatic stress levels and this appeared to be on a continuum between purely cognitive and overly emotional. Empathy is recognised as a somewhat ambiguous construct and one that lacks a universally accepted definition (Regehr et al., 2002; Hojat et al., 2009). The concept is often structured as being on a continuum spanning from cognitive to affective empathy (Gladstein, 1977; Irving & Dickson, 2004). Cognitive empathy is presented as trying to understand the situation from the viewpoint of those affected but adopting this approach can lead to detached analytical behaviours that attempt to convey concern (Rogers, 1957; Irving & Dickson, 2004). Whilst on the other hand affective empathy involves a vicarious emotional connection with those cared for and this connection can leave an emotional residue for the carer (Keefe, 1976).

Hendron (2013) noted that participants with lower emotional intelligence appeared to adopt a much more cognitive approach to dealing with the pain of others, often discussing how they were empathic towards those they cared for and yet their words did not appear to evidence an affective element. This may be one way in which lower emotional intelligence may be beneficial within the secondary traumatisation experience. However, some comments regarding relationships with their parishioners may not be as strong and comments on past and on-going conflicts with parishioners suggests there is a fine balance to be struck between too close an affective connection and the employment of a cognitive approach which may buffer the professional from impact, but may be interpreted by their parishioners as cold and uncaring. This perception may have a knock-on effect within their wider ministry.

In contrast those with high emotional intelligence appear to step beyond what is conceptualised as empathy and potentially into the more mixed waters that include compassion. These individuals spoke of strong emotional connections with those they care for but they also went beyond this and spoke of, at times, feeling responsible for mending situations and alleviating pain and distress. Hardly, surprising this need to mend was a frequent traveller with guilt, especially when the situation was beyond their human capacity to mend. The attitudes of these participants appeared reflective of Neff's (2003) distinction of compassion as the capacity to acknowledge and be moved by the suffering of others and the desire or need to feel you can change the suffering of others. This was a valuable discovery as it opened up several exciting avenues for discussion.

Firstly, in relation to the secondary traumatisation experience, empathy is frequently hailed as a risk factor for negative impact. However, in Hendron's (2013) case, it was not empathy alone that appeared to be a potential factor for impact but what Hendron perceived as compassion. As discussed in previous chapters, Figley (1995) changed the term 'secondary traumatic stress' to 'compassion fatigue' as a less stigmatised label, however he went on to identify empathy, not compassion, as the risk factor. Thus, we can begin to see how this clouds the waters as to what is the actual risk factor? Is it empathy or compassion?

MacRitchie & Leibowitz (2010) remark there remains a lack of studies that focus on the role empathy plays in the transmission of secondary impact and as such the acceptance of empathy as a risk factor remains accepted without being validated. Hendron (2013) points towards the need to perhaps revisit the roots of secondary impact and to step back and examine whether it is the influence of compassion or empathy raising the risk of impact.

Occupations such as counselling and mental heath operate within more clearly defined therapeutic frameworks where empathy is necessary for the therapeutic alliance but the emphasis of responsibility for change and resolution lies firmly within the client's control not the professionals. Therefore, compassion rather than empathy as a risk factor may be a more salient issue for professions such as clergy, which operate outside a distinct therapeutic framework.

Finally, on the topic of empathy Hendron (2013) noted that some lower emotional intelligence participants were somewhat of an anomaly. They appeared to offer less affective connection to those they care for and yet they often spoke of feeling empathic towards tragic situations in the past. In fact for some, the compassionate care of others was a core reason for joining the ministry. Thus, suggesting at one point they were more empathic to what was going on. This led to the consideration that perhaps the impact of trauma work may act as a corrosive element to constructs such as empathy and compassion in some individuals and even further it may erode factors such as emotional intelligence over time.

This is a somewhat unique approach to understanding the concept as it is normally discussed in terms of it being enhanced and developed through training and has not previously been discussed in terms of it decreasing through negative experiences. It is worth noting that although emotional intelligence reducing over time has received no attention, the closely aligned concept of empathy has been shown to erode over time in certain circumstances.

Hojat et al. (2009) carried out a longitudinal study amongst medical students which indicated that whilst empathy did not change during the first two years, it did significantly decrease at the end of third year and this decrease persisted till after graduation. This result carried across gender and medical discipline. Factors attributed to this decrease included realities of patient environment, behaviour of superiors that promoted an uncaring approach and hostile patient environments with a fear of making mistakes. These factors are not dissimilar to those identified by some of Hendron's (2013) participants in relation to their trauma work and as such it is valuable when setting in place support strategies for clergy to consider if emotional intelligence and empathy are being eroded within the challenging environment of the pastoral ministry.

Finally, an important element to be considered in terms of clergy welfare once again emerged from Hendron's (2013) study. Those clergy with higher emotional intelligence afforded themselves self-compassion. Neff (2003) identifies self-compassion as a healthy non-judgemental attitude towards oneself. Heffernan et al. (2010) identified self-compassion as a core component in the ability to be compassionate towards others, suggesting that to provide such self-care one needs to have an objective, realistic view of one's own emotions. These same authors reported a significant association between emotional intelligence as measured by the Trait emotional intelligence questionnaire (Petrides & Furnham, 2003) and self-compassion as measured by the Self Compassion scale (Neff, 2003).

Hendron's (2013) study points towards the associations between higher emotional intelligence facilitating self-compassion not as a selfish indulgence but as an important component in the battle with secondary impact as those who were more caring towards themselves appeared more likely to seek help in an attempt to alleviate how they were feeling, which in turn may also aid in the management of unrealistic expectations of being able to resolve situations and reduce associated feelings of guilt.

Saakvitne & Pearlman (1996) suggest there are three central aspects that need to be present before any intervention to assist in the management of negative impact can be effective. They simplify these aspects into an ABC format.

- **A** represents awareness and reflects the individual's ability and willingness to be attuned to their inner state and to recognise when its balance is disturbed by the force of the work.

- **B** represents balance and reflects the individual's endeavours to maintain a balance between their challenging work and the more positive aspects of their lives. Saakvitne & Pearlman (1996) also contend this involved being able to engage with their inner resources to reflect on what is taking place in order to direct their choices to reinstate equilibrium.

- **C** represents the connections the individual must maintain to themselves and to others around them and to recognise and seek interpersonal resources as a valuable tool to alleviate the impact. Connection also involves being with something larger than them in order to give an anchor for their lives when they are mixed within the chaotic lives of those they help.

Hendron's (2013) findings suggested the benefits of emotional intelligence in undertaking this simple ABC strategy and there emerged a blueprint of higher emotional intelligence effectively facilitating this positive strategy. Maxwell (2005) strongly advocates creating visual conceptualisations in order to help clarify what is taking place. Additionally, Miles & Huberman (1994) state, '*You know what you display*' (p91). Based on these proposals Hendron (2013) devised the visual mnemonic '*H.A.L.O.*' capturing the influence of emotional intelligence upon the recognition and management of secondary impact. This is represented in Figure 1

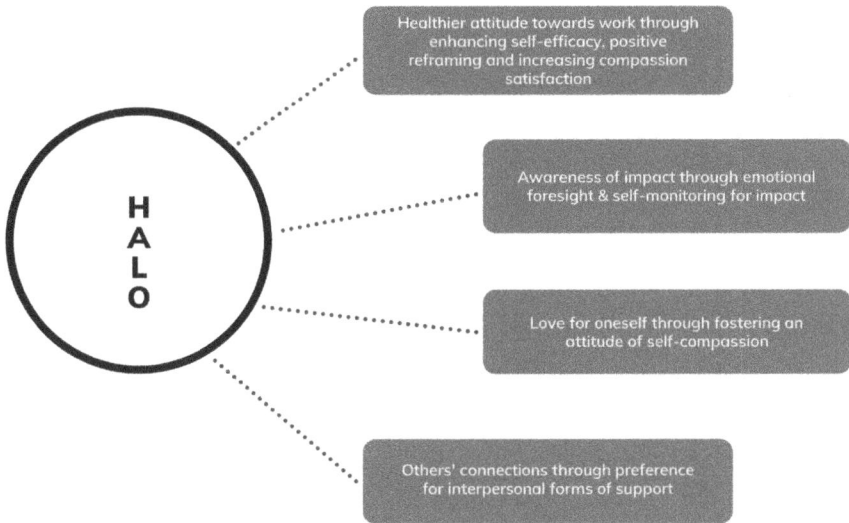

H. A. L. O: Model of the Influence of emotional intelligence within the Recognition & Management of Secondary Impact.

More recently Figely & Figley (2017) introduced the concept of compassion resilience which appears to encompass many of the stands already discussed within this chapter. This they contend is a spectrum of resources that are available to workers within the caring roles that can range from very low resilience to very high. The high resilience end of the spectrum is of particular interest within this chapter as they represent it as consisting of protective factors previously discussed such as self-care, accessing social support and a genuine sense of satisfaction in the work undertaken.

In conclusion, this chapter has attempted to focus on the more positive elements associated with the caring role. It has also endeavoured to introduce emotional intelligence as a factor that is worthy of consideration by both individuals and organisations as tool which could be of central importance for making the experience of caring more positive and enriching.

Chapter 8

Where do we go From Here? Applications for Church Organisations & Individual Clergy

The previous chapters have undertaken an extensive journey through existing understanding of the challenges and rewards of ministerial life and they clearly show that, as the title of this book suggests, at times it can be a painful process to provide this essential care and support. It would now be remiss to conclude this book without setting in place some concise applications that could be adopted by both individual clergy and by those who hold responsibility for their training and support. Therefore, several key factors that were discussed in detail in previous chapters are now set out in concise bullet form.

Firstly, we have unpacked the following in relation to the experience of clergy when working with crisis:

- Secondary impact from trauma does not only emerge from involvement in large scale trauma events but can be a result of a single or multiple encounters with what can appear to the outside observer as minor crisis situations.

- This impact can be both negative and positive in its nature and can present those who experience it with significant personal and professional challenges.

- Clergy are frequently intrinsic support elements within both large and small scale crisis experiences that individuals and communities may encounter. This may take the form of early and long-term crisis assistance.

- Due to the very essence of the ministerial role, clergy present a complex picture and one that requires specific understanding of the co-existence of trauma impact and ministerial responsibilities. These can differ significantly from other trauma support professionals and as such, the training and support provided should acknowledge this and be tailored to the specific characteristics and needs of the ministry.

- The current global Covid-19 pandemic has taken a toll upon us all. Undoubtedly, many clergy have been at the forefront of providing care and support during this period and therefore an additional toll has been placed upon them. The global recovery from this pandemic may possibly take many years and therefore it is highly likely that communities and individuals will continue to look to clergy for emotional and spiritual support.

- Due to the potential trauma exposure that their pastoral ministry presents, clergy need to be both trained and supported for this element of their role.

- The very essence of the pastoral role may predispose clergy to the cost of caring. It is recognised that these cannot be completely removed. Therefore, personal strategies are salient that could assist individuals to positively recognise and manage this cost and emotional intelligence skills may be a personal factor which can positively assist in this process.

On initial consideration, it would be easy to think this paints a fatalistic picture of the ministry wherein the giving of empathy, care and support that the role requires means there is little the individual or the organisation can do to avoid impact. However, this book and the practical ministry experiences and empirical research wherein it was grounded suggest that all is not lost and a number of things can be done on both an organisational and individual level to mediate the impact.

Organisational Level:

- It is imperative that during their initial ministerial training, clergy should be educated to recognise the potential for negative impacts from their pastoral ministry.

- The culture within Church organisations should be one of recognising, and actively promoting wellness as an essential part of the pastoral ministry. This needs to be acknowledged and accepted across the spectrum of those who hold the highest office to individual congregations wherein clergy are placed.

- Organisations should ensure that clergy are made aware of the impact caring work can have in the short term as a natural consequence of their role and can be positively managed. However, without an awareness that this impact can occur, the potential for more negative consequences heightens.

- Training on this concept should be embedded within initial ministerial training and therefore prepare and equip clerics before they become exposed. For those already out working within their own parishes it should be part of a required continuing professional development (CPD) programme of training.

- Be aware that risk factors for clergy may be different from other caring professionals and therefore training should be specifically designed and targeted.

- Educate clergy to recognise the triggers and the signs of impact and to distinguish them from the more general stresses of the ministry.

- Have in place practical self-care protocols for those involved in the pastoral ministry. Ensure that these are clearly articulated and embedded within accepted clergy practices.

- For reasons beyond the scope of this book clergy emotional intelligence appears in general to be low and as such the inclusion of factors such as emotional intelligence training within ordination programmes is worthy of consideration.

- Organisational support networks for clergy should not only be available during times of crisis but should be sufficiently funded to enable proactive engagement with clergy on a regular basis to ensure their wellbeing is valued and supported.

Individual Level:

In terms of personal responsibility for their own wellbeing, there are a number of factors that clergy can consider to provide protection and support. For simplicity of recall and ease of adoption it is worthwhile revisiting the acronym of H.A.L.O previously discussed in detail in Chapter 7. The steps that H.A.L.O set are key to clergy ensuring that they embed a positive wellness protocol into their ministerial role.

- **H: Healthier attitude**. Remain open to embracing wellbeing as an essential part of their lives and ministries and recognise it as something that has a high value, requiring self-compassion and personal investment.

- **A: Awareness of impact:** Clergy should adopt an attitude of personal responsibility for monitoring impacts from specific elements of their role. Individuals should practice self-exploration and reflection whereby they can identify and understand any specific factors or experiences that may present as particularly challenging for them personally. Given that at times the impact from these encounters is not personally recognised, clergy should consider having an accountability colleague who is both a form of support and is permitted to point out any issues that may emerge.

- **L: Love of oneself**: View self-care and self-compassion as essential and ethical requirements of their ministry rather than a form of self-indulgence for those who have the time to be retrospective. Set personal and professional boundaries and goals that are healthy, realistic and achievable.

- **O: Other's Connections:** Keep open connections with others as, for a number of reasons, ministerial life can be a lonely and the bounds of confidentiality associated with many crisis situations can leave clergy alone with thoughts and emotions that require exploration and processing. Recognise that working alone can lead to feelings of isolation and lack of support. Demanding vestries and parishioners with unrealistic expectations can result in being unable to acknowledge impact and seek the essential support required. At times, we all require the support, compassion and love of others to get us through tough episodes. Building up good personal support networks is essential and should be adopted from the point of initial training. The availability of professional, confidential support should be accessed without embarrassment or detrimental professional consequences.

In closing as the tile of this book suggests, for many clergy it hurts to care and as this book has articulated, the very essence of the pastoral ministry means factors that evoke this hurt will be encountered. However, this should not mean that individual clergy and those who hold responsibility for their welfare should not do everything within their power to help this to hurt a little less.

REFERENCES

Abendroth, M. & Flannery, J. (2006). Predicting the risk of compassion fatigue: study of hospice nurses, *Journal of Hospice and Palliative Nursing,* 8, 346–356.

Abernethy, A. (2002). *Fulfillment and frustration: ministry in today's church.* Blackrock: The Columba Press.

Adams, K.B., Matto, H.C. & Harrington, D. (2001). The Traumatic Stress Institute Belief Scale as a measure of vicarious trauma in a national sample of clinical social workers. *Families in Society: The Journal of Contemporary Human Services,* 82, 363-371.

Adams, N. (1995). Spirituality, science and therapy. *Australian and New Zealand Journal of Family Therapy,* 16(4), 201-208.

Adams, R.E., Figley, C.R. & Boscarino, J. A. (2008). The Compassion Fatigue Scale: its uses with social workers following urban disaster. *Research on Social Work Practice,* 18, 238-250.

Akerjordet, K. & Severinsson, E. (2004). Emotional Intelligence in mental health nurses talking about practice. *International Journal of Mental Health Nursing,* 13,164-170.

Akerjordet, K. & Severinsson, E. (2007). Emotional Intelligence; a review of the literature with specific focus on empirical and epistemological perspectives. *Journal of Clinical Nursing,* 16,1405-1416.

Akerjordet, K. & Severinsson, E. (2009). Emotional Intelligence and nursing: A integrative literature review. *International Journal of Nursing Studies,* 46(12), 1624-1636.

Allt, J. (1999). Vicarious trauma: a survey of clinical counselling psychologists. Unpublished doctoral dissertation. England: University of Surrey.

American Psychiatric Association. (1987). *Diagnostic and Statistical Manual of Mental Disorders.* (3rd ed., rev. Washington, DC: Author

American Psychiatric Association (2000). *Diagnostic and Statistical Manual of Mental Disorders.* 4th ed. revision. Washington, DC: Author.

American Psychiatric Association (2013). *Diagnostic and Statistical Manual of Mental Disorders.* 5th ed. revision. Washington, DC: Author.

Argyle, M. & Lu, L. (1990). The happiness of extraverts. *Personality & Individual Differences,* 11, 1011-1017.

Arnold, D., Calhoun, L.G. Tedeschi, R. & Cann, A. (2005). Vicarious posttraumatic growth in psychotheraphy. *Journal of Humanistic Psychology,* 45(2), 239-263.

Arvay, M.J. (2001). Secondary traumatic stress among trauma counsellors: what does the research say? *International Journal for the Advancement of Counselling,* 23(4), 283-293.

Arvay, M.J. & Uhlemann, M.R. (1996). Counsellor stress and impairment in the field of trauma. *The Canadian Journal of Counselling,* 30(3),193-210.

Austin, E.J., Evans, P., Magnus, B & O'Hanlon, K. (2007). A preliminary study of empathy, emotional intelligence and examination performance in MBChB students. *Medical Education,* 41, 684-689.

Azizian, S. & Samadi, I. (2012). Study of relationship between Emotional Intelligence (EI) and self-efficacy the case of the staff of the Hamedan Branch of the Islamic Azad University. *Procedia-Social & Behavioral Sciences,* 31, 496-502.

Bach, M. & Bach, D. (1995). Predictive value of alexithymia: a prospective study in somatizing patients. *Psychotherapy & Psychomatics,* 64, 43-48.

Baird, S. & Jenkins, S.R. (2003). Vicarious traumatization, secondary traumatic stress and burnout in sexual assault and domestic violence agency staff. *Violence and Victims,*18, 71-85.

Baird, K. & Kracen, A.C. (2006). Vicarious traumatization and secondary traumatic stress: a research synthesis. *Counseling Psychology Quarterly,* 19(2), 181-188.

Bandura, A., Capprara, G.V, Barbaranelli, C., Gerbino, M. & Pasorelli, C. (2003). Role of affective self-regulatory efficacy in diverse spheres of psychological functioning. *Child Development,* 74, 769-782.

Barna, G. (1999). *Highly effective churches.* Ventura: Issachar Resources.

Barnsteiner, J.H. & Gillis-Donovan, J. (1990). Being related and separate: a standard for therapeutic relationships. *American Journal of Maternal Child Nursing,* 15, 223-228.

Bates, K.M. (2005*). Moderators for secondary traumatic stress in human services professionals: the role of emotional, cognitive and social factors.* Capella University. Available from Proquest http://proquest.umi.com/pqdlink [Accessed 9 January 2010]

Beaton, R. & Murphy, S.A. (1995). Working people in crisis: research implications. In C.R. Figley (Ed.) *Compassion Fatigue. Coping with secondary PTSD among those who treat the traumatized.* New York: Brunner Mazel.

Beaumont, S. (2011). Pastoral counseling down under: a survey of Australian clergy. *Pastoral Psychology* 60(1), 117-131.

Beck, C.T. & Gable, R.K. (2012). A Mixed Methods study of Secondary Traumatic Stress in Labor and Delivery Nurses. *Journal of Obstretric Gynecologic & Neonatal Nursing,* Jul 12. doi: 10.1111/j.1552-6909.2012.01386..x. Available at: http://www.ncbi.nlm.nih.gov/pubmed/22788967 [Accessed 4 August 2012]

Beebe, R.S. (2007). Predicting Burnout, Conflict Management Style and Turnover Among Clergy. *Journal of Career Assessment,* 15(2), 257-275.

Bell, H. (2003). Strengths and secondary trauma in family violence work. *Social Work,* 48(4), 513-522.

Ben-Porat, A. & Itzhaky, H. (2009). Implication of treating family violence for the therapist: secondary traumatization, vicarious traumatization and growth. *Journal of Family Violence,* 24, 507-515.

Benight, C.C. & Harper, M.L. (2002). Coping self-efficacy perceptions as a mediator between acute stress response and long-term distress following natural disasters. *Journal of Traumatic Stress,* 15, 177-186.

Benoit, L.G. Veach, P.M. & LeRoy, B.S. (2007). When you care enough to do your best: genetic counselor experiences of compassion fatigue. *Journal of Genetic Counseling,* 16 (3), 299-312.

Berry, A., Francis, L.J., Rolph, J. & Rolph, P. (2012). Ministry and stress: listening to Anglican clergy in Wales. *Pastoral Psychology,* 61,165-178.

Black, S. & Weinreich, P. (2001). An exploration of counseling identity in counselors who deal with trauma. *Traumatology,* 7, 85-90.

Bober, T. & Regehr, C. (2006). Strategies for reducing secondary or vicarious trauma: Do they work? *Brief Treatment and Crisis Intervention,* 6(1), 1-9.

Boscarino, J.A., Figley, C.R. & Adams, R.E. (2004). Compassion fatigue following the September 11 terrorist attacks: a study of secondary trauma among New York city social workers. *International Journal of Emergency Mental Health,* 6(2), 57-66.

Boyatzis, R.E., Brizz, T. & Godwin, L.N. (2011). The Effect of Religious Leaders' Emotional and Social Competencies on Improving Parish Vibrancy. *Journal of Leadership & Organizational Studies,* 18(2), 192-206.

Boyer, B.A., Knolls, M.L., Kafkalas, C.M., Tollen, L. G., & Swartz, M. (2000). Prevalence and relationships of posttraumatic stress in families experiencing pediatric spinal cord injury. *Rehabilitation Psychology, 45,* 339-355.

Bradfield, C., Wylie, M.L., and Echterling, L.G. (1989). After the flood: The response of ministers to a natural disaster. *Sociological Analysis,* 49(4), 397-407.

Brady, J., Guy, J., Poelstra, P. & Brokaw, B. (1999). Vicarious traumatisation, spirituality and the treatment of sexual abuse survivors: a national survey of women psychotherapists. *Professional Psychology Research & Practice,* 30, 386-393.

Bride, B.E., Radey, M., & Figley, C. (2007). Measuring Compassion Fatigue. *Clinical Social Work Journal,* 35(3), 155-163.

Bride, B.E., Robinson, M.M., Yegidis, B. & Figley, C.R. (2003). Development and validation of the Secondary Traumatic Stress Scale. *Research on Social Work Practice,* 13, 1-16.

Buchanan, M., Anderson, J.O. Uhlemann, M.B. & Horwitz. M.J. (2006). Secondary traumatic stress: an investigation of Canadian mental health workers. *Traumatology,* 12(4), 272-281.

Burton, J. & Burton, C. (2009). *Public people, private lives: tackling stress in clergy families.* London: Continuum.

Camerlengo, H. (2002). *The role of coping style, job-related stress, and personal victimization history in the vicarious traumatization of professional who work with abused youth.* Unpublished doctoral dissertation. New Jersey; Rutgers University.

Caruso, D. & Salovey, P. (2004). *The Emotionally Intelligent Manager.* San Francisco: Jossey-Base.

Case, A.D., Keyes, C.L.M., Huffman, K.F., Sittser, K., Wallace, A., Khatiwoda, P., Parnell, H.E., & Proeschold-Bell, R.J. (2020) Attitudes and behaviors that differentiate clergy with positive mental health from those with burnout, *Journal of Prevention & Intervention in the Community,* 48:1, 94-112

Catherall, D.R. (1995). Coping with secondary traumatic stress: the importance of the therapist's professional peer group. In B.H. Stamm (Ed.) *Secondary traumatic stress: self-care issues for clinicians, researchers and educators*. (pp. 29-36) Lutherville, MD: Sidran

Chamberlain, J. & Miller, M.K. (2009). Evidence of secondary traumatic stress, safety concerns and burnout among a homogeneous group of judges in a single jurisdiction. *Journal of The American Academy of Psychiatry and the Law*, 37(2), 212-224.

Chandler, D.J. (2009). Pastoral burnout and the impact of personal spiritual renewal, rest taking, and support systems practice. *Pastoral Psychology*, 58, 273-287.

Charlton, R., Rolph, J., Francis, L.J., Rolph, P. & Robbbins, M. (2009). Clergy work-related psychological health: listening to the ministers of the word and sacrament within the United Reformed Church in England. *Pastoral Psychology*, 58, 133-149.

Chinnici, R. (1985). Pastoral care following a natural disaster. *Pastoral Psychology*, 33(4), 245-254.

Chrestman, K.R. (1995). Secondary exposure to trauma and self-reported distress amongst therapists. In B.H. Stamm (Ed.) *Secondary traumatic stress: self-care for clinicians, researchers and educators* (pp. 29-36). Lutherville, MD: Sidran Press.

Church of England (2011). *Experiences in Ministry Project: Respondents findings report*. Available from http://www.experiencesofministry.org/ [Accessed 20 January 2012].

Ciarrochi, J., Deane, F. P. & Anderson, S. (2002). Emotional Intelligence Moderates the Relationship Between Stress and Mental Health. *Personality & Individual Differences*, 32, 197–209.

Ciarrochi, J. & Scott, G. (2006). The link between emotional competence and well-being: a longitudinal study. *British Journal of Guidance & Counselling*, 34(2), 231-243.

Cohen, M.S. (1989). The rabbi and the holocaust survivor. In P. Marcus & A. Rosenberg (Eds.) *Healing their wounds: psychotherapy with Holocaust survivors and their families* (pp. 167-176). New York: Prageer.

Cole, A.H. Jr. (2010). What makes care pastoral? *Pastoral Psychology*, 59, 711-723.

Collins, S. & Long, A. (2003). Too tired to care? The psychological effects of working with trauma. *Journal of Psychiatric and Mental Health Nursing*, 10(1) 17-27.

Conrad, D. & Kellar-Guenther, Y. (2006). Compassion fatigue, burnout and compassion satisfaction among Colorado child protection workers. *Child Abuse & Neglect*, 30(10), 1071-1080.

Cooper, A.E. (2003). An investigation of the relationships among spirituality, prayer, and meditation, and aspects of stress and coping. *Dissertation Abstracts International* (UMI no. 3084474).

Craig, C.D. & Sprang, G. (2010). Compassion satisfaction, compassion fatigue and burnout in a national sample of trauma treatment therapists. *Anxiety Stress & Coping*, 23(3), 319-339.

Cranfield, J. (2005). Secondary Traumatisation, Burnout, and Vicarious Traumatisation: A Review of the Literature as it Relates to Therapists who Treat Trauma. *Smith College Studies in Social Work*, 75(2): 81–102.

Creamer, T.L. (2002). *Secondary trauma and coping processes among mental health workers responding to the September 11 attacks*. Unpublished doctoral dissertation. Auburn University.

Crisp-Han, H., Gabbard, G.O. & Martinez, M. (2011). Professional boundary violation and mentalizing in the clergy. *Journal of Pastoral Care & Counseling*, 65(3), 1-11.

Crossley, K. (2002). Professional satisfaction among US healthcare chaplains. *Journal of Pastoral Care & Counseling*, 56(1), 1-7.

Crothers, D. (1995). Vicarious traumatization in the work with survivors of childhood trauma. *Journal of Psychosocical Nursing Mental Health Services* 33(4), 9-13.

Croucher, R. (1991). *Recent trends amongst evangelicals: Biblical agenda, justice and spirituality*. Victoria: John Mark Ministries.

Csiernik, R. & Adams, D.W. (2002). Spirituality, stress and work. *Employee Assistance Quarterly*, 18(2), 29-37.

Cunningham, M. (2003). Impact of trauma work on social work clinicians: Empirical findings. *Social Work*, 48, 451-459.

Dane, B. (2000). Child welfare workers: an innovative approach for interacting with secondary trauma. *Journal of Social Work Education*, 36, 27-38.

Darling, C.A., Hill, E.W. & McWey, L.M. (2004). Understanding stress and quality of life for clergy and clergy spouses. *Stress & Health*, 20, 261-277.

Dekel, R., Hantman, S., Ginzburg, K & Solomon, Z. (2006). The cost of caring? Social workers in hospital confront ongoing terrorism. *British Journal of Social Work*, 37, 1247-1261.

Devilly, G., Wright, R. & Vaker, T. (2009). Vicarious trauma, secondary traumatic stress or simply burnout? Effects of trauma therapy on mental health professionals. *Australian & New Zealand Journal of Psychiatry*, 43(4), 373-385.

Dickes, S.J. (1998). *Treating sexually abused children versus adults: an exploration of secondary traumatic stress and vicarious traumatization among therapists.* Unpublished doctoral dissertation. Frenso: California School of Professional Psychology.

Doolittle, B.R. (2007). Burnout and coping amongst parish-based clergy. *Mental Health, Religion & Coping*, 10(1), 31-38.

Dunkley, J. & Whelan, T.A. (2006). Vicarious traumatisation in telephone counsellors; internal and external influences. *British Journal of Counselling*, 34(4), 451-469.

Dunn, E.W., Brackett, M.A., Ashton-James, C., Schneiderman, E. & Salovey, P. (2007). On Emotionally Intelligent Time Travel: Individual Differences in Affective Forecasting Ability. *PSPB*, 33(1), 85-93.

Dyregrov, A. & Mitchell, J.T. (1996). Work with traumatized clients: psychological effects and coping strategies. *Journal of Traumatic Stress*, 5, 5-17.

Ebear, J., Csiernik, R. & Bechard, M. (2008). Furthering parish wellness: including social work as part of a Catholic pastoral team. *Social Work & Christianity*, 35(2), 179-196.

Ehlers, A., Clark, D.M., Hackman, A., Grey, N., Lineos, S., Wild, J., Manley, J., Waddington, L. & McManus, F. (2010). Intensive cognitive therapy for PTSD: a feasibility study. *Behavioural & Cognitive Psychotherpy*, 38(40), 383-398.

Engstrom, D., Hernandez, P. & Gangsei, D. (2008). Vicarious resilience: a qualitative investigation into its description. *Traumatology*, 14(3), 13-21.

Epstein, S. (1985). The implication of cognitive-experiential self-theory for research in social psychology and personality. *Journal for the Theory of Social Behavior*, 15, 283-310.

Everly, G.S. Jr. (2000). The role of pastoral crisis intervention in disasters, terrorism, violence and other community crisis. *International Journal of Emergency Mental Health*, 2(3), 139-142.

Extremera, N. & Fernández-Berrocal, P. (2005). Perceived emotional intelligence and life satisfaction: predictive and incremental validity using trait Meta-Mood Scale. *Personality and Individual Differences*, 39, 937-948.

Farrrell, J.L. & Goebert, D.A. (2008). Collaboration between psychiatrists and clergy in recognizing and treating serious mental illness. *Psychiatric Services*, 59(4), *437-440.*

Feldman, D. B., & Kaal, K. J. (2007). Vicarious trauma and assumptive worldview: Beliefs about the world in acquaintances of trauma victims. *Traumatology*, 3, 21-31.

Figley, C.R. (1978). *Stress disorders amongst Vietnam veterans.* New York: Brunner/Mazel.

Figley, C.R. (1983). Catastrophe: An overview of family reactions. In C.R. Figley & H.I. McCubbin (Eds). *Stress and the family: vol 2. Coping with catastrophe* (pp. 3-20). New York: Brunner/Mazel.

Figley, C.R (1989). *Helping traumatized famlilies.* San Francisco, CA: Jossey-Bass.

Figley, C.R. (1993). *Trauma and its wake. (Vol 2). Traumatic stress, theory, research and intervention.* New York: Brunner/Mazel.

Figley, C.R. (1995). *Compassion fatigue: coping with Secondary Traumatic Stress Disorder in those who threat the traumatized.* New York: Brunner/Mazel.

Figley, C.R. (1996). Review of the Compassion Fatigue Self-Test. In B.H. Stamm (Ed.) *Measurement of stress, trauma and adaption.* Baltimore, MD: Sidran Press.

Figley, C.R. (1999). Compassion fatigue: towards a new understanding of the cost of caring. In B.H. Stamm (Ed.) *Secondary traumatic stress: self-care issues for clinicians, researchers and educators.* 2nd Ed. Lutherville, MD: Sidran Press.

Figley, C.R. (2002a). *Treating compassion fatigue.* New York: Brunner/Routledge.

Figley, C.R. (2002b). Compassion Fatigue. Psychotherapists' chronic lack of self -care. *Journal of Clinical Practice*, 8, 1433-1441.

Figley CR, Figley KR. Compassion fatigue resilience. In: Seppälä EM, Simons-Thomas E, Brown SL, Worline MC, Cameron CD, Doty JR, editors. *The Oxford handbook of compassion science.* New York: Oxford University Press; 2017. p. 387–98.

Figley, C.R. & Roop, R. (2006). *Compassion fatigue in the animal care community.* Washington, DC: Humane Society Press.

Finch, J. (1983). *Married to the job.* London: Alllen & Unwin.

Flannelly, K.J., Roberts, S.B. & Weaver, A.J. (2005). Correlates of compassion fatigue and burnout in chaplains and other clergy who responded to the September 11th attacks in New York City. *The Journal of Pastoral Care & Counseling*, 59(3), 213-224.

Flannelly, K.J., Weaver, A.J. Smith, W.J. & Oppenheimer, J.E. (2003). A systematic review on chaplains and community-based clergy in three palliative care journals: 1990-1999. *American Journal of Hospital Palliative Care*, 20, 263-268.

Fletcher, B. (1990). *Clergy under stress*. London: Mowbray.

Flier, L.L. (1995). "Demystifying mysticism: Finding a developmental relationship between different ways of knowing". *The Journal of Transpersonal Psychology*, 27(2), 131-152.

Foa, E., Riggs, D. & Dancu, C. (1993). Reliability and validity of a brief instrument for assessing posttraumatic stress disorder, *Journal of Trauma Stress*, 6, 459–473.

Follette, M., Polusny, V. & Milbeck, K. (1994). Mental health and law enforcement professionals: trauma history, psychological symptoms, and the impact of providing services to child sexual abuse survivors. *Professional Psychological Research*, 25, 275-282.

Francis, L.J., Hills, P. & Kaldor, P. (2009). The Oswald Clergy Burnout Scale: reliability, factor structure and preliminary application among Australian clergy. *Pastoral Psychology*, 57, 243-252.

Francis, L.J. & Lankshear, D. (1992). The Catholic Evangelical consensus: a study on attitudes of the clergy. *Contact*, 108, 17-22.

Francis, L.J., Louden, S.H. & Rutledge, C.J.F. (2004). Burnout among Roman Catholic Parochial Clergy in England and Wales: Myth or Reality? *Review of Religious Research*, 46(1), 5-19.

Francis, L.J., Robbins, M., Kaldor, P. & Castle, K. (2009). Psychological type and work-related psychological health among clergy in Australia, England and New Zealand. *Journal of Psychology and Christianity*, 28(3), 200-212.

Francis, L.J., & Rutledge, C.J.F. (2000). Are rural clergy in the Church of England under greater stress? A study in empirical theology. *Research in the Social Scientific Study of Religion, 11*, 173-191.

Francis, L.J., Ryland, A. & Robbins, M. (2011). Emotional Intelligence among church leaders: applying The Schutte Emotional Intelligence Scale within Newfrontiers. In Boag, S. & Tiliopoulos, N. (Eds.) *Personality & Individual Differences: Theory, assessment, & application*. New York: Nova Science Publishers.

Francis, L.J. & Turton, D.W. (2004). Recognising and understanding burnout among clergy: a perspective from empirical theology. In D. Herl & M.L. Berman (Eds.) *Building bridges over troubled waters: enhancing pastoral care and guidance* (pp. 307-331). Lima, OH: Wyndham Hall Press.

Francis, L.J., Wulff, K. & Robbins, M. (2008). The relationship between work-related psychological health and psychological type amongst clergy serving in the Presbyterian Church (USA). *Journal of Empirical Theology*, 21, 166-182.

Frese, M. (1999). Social support as a moderator of the relationship between work stressors and psychological dysfunctioning. *Journal of Occupational Health Psychology*, 4(3), 179-192.

Freud, A. (1969). Comments on psychic trauma. *In the Writings of Anna Freud. Vol. 5*, 221-241. New York: International Universities Press.

Freudenberger, H. (1974). Staff burnout. *Journal of Social Issues*, 30, 159-165

Funder, D.C (2001). Personality. *Annual Review of Psychology*, 52,197-221.

Furr, R.M. & Funder, D.C. (1998). A multimodal analysis of personal negativity. *Personality & Social Psychology*, 74, 1580-1591.

Galek, K., Flannelly, K.J., Green, P.B. & Kudler, T. (2011). Burnout, secondary traumatic stress and social support. *Pastoral Psychology*, 60, 633-649.

Gallup, G. & Lindsay, D.M. (1999). *Surveying the religious landscape: Trends in U.S. beliefs*. Harrisburg, PA: Morehouse.

Garter, J., Larson, D.B. & Allen, G.D. (1991). Religious commitment and mental health: a review of the empirical literature. *Journal of Psychology & Theology*,19(1), 6-25.

Genia, V. & Shaw, D. G. (1991). Religion, Intrinsic extrinsic orientation and depression. *Review of Religious Research*, 32, 274-283.

Gentry, J.E. (2002). Compassion fatigue. A crucible of transformation. *Journal of Trauma Practice*, 1(3), 37-61.

Gentry, J.E., Baggerly, J. & Baranowsky, A. (2004). Training-as-treatment: effectiveness of the Certified Compassion Fatigue Specialist Training. *International Journal of Emergency Mental Health*, 6(3), 147-155.

George, J.M. (1995). Leader positive mood and group performance: the case of customer service. *Journal of Applied Social Psychology*, 25, 778-794.

Ghahramanlou, M. & Brodbeck, C. (2000). Predictors of secondary trauma in sexual assault trauma counselors. *International Journal of Emergency Mental Health*, 2, 229-240.

Gibson, M. & Iwaniec, D. (2003). An empirical study into the psychosocial reactions of staff working as helpers to those affected by two traumatic incidents. *British Journal of Social Work*, 33, 851-870.

Gillman, J., Gable-Rodriquez, J., Sutherland, M. & Whitacre, J. (1996). Pastoral Care in a Critical Care Setting. *Critical Care Nursing Quarterly*, 19, 10-20.

Gladstein, G.A. (1977). Empathy and the counseling outcome: an empirical and conceptual review. *The Professional Forum*, 6(4), 70-79.

Goffman, I. (1963). *Stigma: notes on the management of spoiled identity.* London: Penguin Books.

Gooch, S. (2006). Emotionally smart. *Nursing standards,* 20, 20-22.

Graham, S., Furr, S., Flowers, C. & Burke, M.T. (2001). Religion and spirituality in coping with stress. *Counseling and Values*, 46(1), 2-14.

Grosh, W.N. & Olsen, D.C. (2000). Clergy burnout: an integrative approach. *Psychology in Practice,* 56(5), 619-632.

Gross, J.J. (2002). Emotion regulation: affective, cognitive and social consequences. *Psychotherapy*, 39, 281-291.

Hang-yue, N., Foley, S. & Loi, R. (2005). Work role stressors and turnover intentions: a study of professional clergy in Hong Kong. *The International Journal of Human Resource Management,* 16(11), 2133-2146.

Harrison, R.L. & Westwood, M.J. (2009). Preventing vicarious traumatization of mental health therapists: identifying protective practices. *Psychotherapy*, 46(2), 203-219.

Heffernan, M., Griffin, M.T.Q., McNulty, R. & Fitzpatrick, J.J. (2010). Self-compassion and Emotional Intelligence in nurses. *International Journal of Nursing Practice,* 16, 366-373.

Hemmelgarn, A. L., Glisson, C. & James, L. R. (2006). Organizational culture and climate: Implications for services and interventions research. *Clinical Psychology: Science and Practice,* 13, 73-89.

Hendron, J.A. (2013) *The secondary traumatisation experience of Church of Ireland clergy and its relationship with emotional intelligence.* PhD. Thesis. Ulster University

Hendron, J.A., Irving, P. & Taylor, B. (2012). The unseen cost: a discussion of the secondary traumatization experience of clergy. *Pastoral Psychology,* 61(2), 221-231.

Herman, J.L. (1992). *Trauma and recovery.* New York: Basic Books.

Hernández, P., Gangsei, D. & Engstrom, D. (2007). Vicarious resilience: a new concept in work with those who survive trauma. *Family Process*, 46(2), 226-241.

Hill, W., Darling, C.A. & Raimondi, N. (2003). Understanding boundary related stress issues in clergy families. *Marriage & Family Review*, 35, 45-62.

Hills, P.J., Francis, L.J. & Rutledge, C.J.F. (2004). The factor structure of a measure of burnout specific to clergy, and its trial application with respect to some individual personal differences. *Review of Religious Research*, 46(1), 27-42.

Hohnman, A.A. & Larson, D.B. (1993). Psychiatric factors predicting the use of clergy. In E.L. Worthington Jr (Ed.) *Psychology and religious values* (pp. 71-84). Grand Rapids, Michigan: Baker Books.

Hojat, M., Vergare, M.J., Maxwell, K., Brainard, G., Herrine, S.K., Isenberg, G.A., Veloski, J. & Gonnella, J. S. (2009). The devil is in the third year: a longitudinal study of erosion of empathy in medical school. *Academic Medicine: the journal of the Association of Medical Colleges*, 84(9), 1182-1191.

Holaday, M., Lackey, T., Boucher, M. & Glidewell, R. (2001). Secondary stress, burnout and the clergy. *American Journal of Pastoral Counselling*, 4(1),53-72.

Holtz, T.H., Salama, P, Cardozo, B.L. & Gotway, C.A. (2002). Mental health status of human rights workers, Kosovs, June 2000. *Journal of Traumatic Stress*, 15(5), 389-395

Hooper, C., Craig, J., Janvrin, D.R., Wetsel., M.A. & Reimels, E. (2010). Compassion satisfaction, burnout and compassion fatigue among emergency nurses compared with nurses in other selected inpatient specialities. *Journal of Emergency Nursing*, 36(5), 420-427.

Horowitz, M.J. (1976). *Stress response syndromes.* Northvale NJ: Aronson Hochschild, A. 1983. The Managed Heart: Commercialization of Human Feeling, Berkeley: University of California Press.

Hunt, N. & Evans, D. (2004). Predicting traumatic stress using Emotional Intelligence. *Behaviour Research & Therapy*, 42(7), 791-798.

Hunter, S.V. & Schofield, M.J. (2006). How counselors cope with traumatized clients: personal, professional and organizational strategies. *International Journal for the Advancement of Counselling*, 28(2), 121-138.

Iliffe, G. & Steed, L.G. (2000). Exploring the counselor's experience of working with perpetrators and survivors of domestic violence. *Journal of Interpersonal Violence*, 15, 393-412.

Imai, H., Nakao, H., Tsuchiya, M., Kuroda, Y & Katon, T. (2004). Burnout and work environments of public health workers involved in mental health care. *Occupational and Environmental Medicine*, 61, 764-768.

Irving, P. & Dickson, D. (2004). Empathy: towards a conceptual framework for health professionals. *International Journal of Health Care Quality Assurance*, 17(4), 212-220.

Isen, A.M. (2001). An Influence of Positive Affect on Decision Making in Complex Situations: Theoretical Issues with Practical Implications. *Journal of Consumer Psychology*, 11(2), 75-85.

Jacob, M. (1983). Post-traumatic stress disorder: facing futility in and after Vietnam. *Currents in Theology and Mission*, 10(5), 291-298

Jacobson, J.M. (2006). Compassion fatigue, compassion satisfaction and burnout. *Journal of Workplace Behavioral* Health, 21(3-4), 133-152.

Jaffe. P.G., Crooks C.V., Dunford-Jackson, B.L. & Town, M. (2006). Vicarious trauma in judges; the personal challenge of dispensing justice. *Judges Journal*, 45(4), 12-18.

Jankowski, R.B., Handzo, G.F. & Flannelly, K.J. (2011). Testing the efficacy of chaplaincy care. *Journal of Health Care Chaplaincy*, 17, 100-125.

Janoff-Bulman, R. (1985). The aftermath of victimization: rebuilding shattered assumptions. In Figley, C.R. (Ed.) *Trauma and its wake: the study and treatment of post-traumatic stress disorder*. New York: Brunner/Mazel.

Jenkins, R.A. & Pargament, K.I. (1995). Religion and spirituality as resources for coping with cancer. *Journal for Psychosocial Oncology*, 13, (1-2), 51-74.

Jenkins, S.R. & Baird, S. (2002). Secondary Traumatic Stress and Vicarious Trauma: a validation study. *Journal of Traumatic Stress*, 15(5), 423-432.

Joinson, C. (1992). Coping with compassion fatigue. *Nursing*, 22 (4), 116-122.

Jordan, P.J., Ashkanasy, N.M. & Härtel, C.E.J. (2002). Emotional intelligence as a moderator of emotional and behavioral reactions to job insecurity. *Academy of Management Review*, 27, 361-372.

Joshi, S., Kumari, S., & Jain, M. (2008). Religious belief and its relationship to psychological wellbeing. *Journal of the Indian Academy of Applied Psychology*, 34(2), 344-354.

Kadambi, M. (2004). Counseling and the professional: vicarious trauma, burnout and the rewards from clinical practice. *Dissertation Abstract International Bulletin Scientific Engineering*, 65(1b), 441.

Kafetsios, K. & Zampetakis, L.A. (2008). Emotional Intelligence and job satisfaction: testing the mediating role of positive and negative affect at work. *Personality & Individual Differences*, 44, 712-722.

Kaldor, P. & Bullpitt, R. (2001). *Burnout in church leaders*. Adelaide, S.S.: Openbook.

Kassai, S.C. & Motta, R. W. (2006). An investigation of potential Holocaust-related secondary traumatization in the third generation. *International Journal of Emergency Mental Health*, 8, 35–47.

Kassam-Adams, N. (1995). The risks of treating sexual trauma: Stress and secondary trauma in psychotherapists. In B.H. Stamm (Ed.) *Secondary traumatic stress; self-care issues for clinicians' researchers and educators* (pp. 37-50). Lutervill, MD: Sidran Press.

Keefe, T. (1976). Empathy: the critical skill. *Social Work*, 21(1), 10-14.

Kemery, E.R. (2006). Clergy role stress and satisfaction: role ambiguity isn't always bad. *Pastoral Psychology*, 54(6), 561-570.

Killlian, K.D. (2008). Helping till it hurts? A multimethod study of compassion fatigue, burnout, and self-care in clinicians working with trauma survivors. *Traumatology*, 14(2), 32-44.

Kinman, G., McFall, O.& Rodriguez, J. (2011). The cost of caring? Emotional labour, wellbeing and the clergy. *Pastoral Psychology*, 60(5), 671-680.

Koenig, H.G. (1992). Religious coping and depression amongst elderly, hospitalized, medically ill men. *American Journal of Psychiatry*, 149(12), 1693-1700.

Koenig, H.G., Larson, D.B., & Larson, S.S. (2001). Religion and coping with serious medical illness. *The Annals of Pharmacotherapy*, 35(3), 352–359.

Kusche, C.A. & Greenberg, M.T. (2001). PATHS in your classroom: Promoting emotional literacy and alleviating emotional distress. In J. Cohen (Ed.), *Social emotional learning and the elementary school child: A guide for educators* (pp. 140–161). New York: Teachers College Press.

Kwako, L.A., Szanton, S.J., Saligan, L.N. & Gill, J.M. (2011). Major Depressive Disorder in Persons Exposed to Trauma: Relationship Between Emotional Intelligence and Social Support. *Journal of the American Psychiatric Nurses Association*, 17(3), 237-245.

Laposa, J. & Alden, M. (2005). Posttraumatic stress disorder in the emergency room: exploration of a cognitive model, *Behaviour Research and Therapy*, 41, 49–65.

Leach, J. & Patterson, M. (2010). *Pastoral supervision*. London: SCM Press

Leavey, G. (2008). UK Clergy and People in mental distress: community and patterns of pastoral care. *Transcultural Psychiatry*, 45(1), 79-104.

Leavey, G., Loewenthal, K. & King, M. (2007). Challenges to sanctuary: the clergy as a resource for mental health care in the community. *Social Science & Medicine*, 65, 548-559.

Lee, C. (2007). Patterns of stress and support amongst Adventist clergy: do pastors and their spouses differs? *Pastoral Psychology*, 55, 761-771.

Lee, R.S. (1980) *Principles of pastoral counselling*. London: SPCK.

Leinweber, J. & Rowe, H.J. (2010). The costs of 'being with the woman': secondary traumatic stress in midwifery. *Midwifery*, 26(1), 76-87.

Lekkos, P. (2008). The risks of vicarious trauma for social work professionals. *Professional Social Work*, Aug,10.

Lepore, S.J., Ragan, J., & Jones, S. (2000). Talking facilitates cognitive-emotional processes of adaption to an acute stressor. *Journal of Personality and Social Psychology*, 78(3), 499-508.

Lepore, S.J. & Smith, J. (2002). (Eds) *The writing cure: how expressive writing influences health and well-being*. Washington, DC: American Psychological Association.

Lerias, D. & Bryne, M.K. (2003). Vicarious traumatization: symptoms and predictors. *Stress & Health*, 19, 129-138.

Lernoux, P. (1980). *Cry of the people*. Garden City, NJ: Doubleday.

Lev-Wiesel, R., Goldblatt, H., Eisikovits, Z. & Admi, H. (2009). Growth in the shadow of war: the case of social workers and nurses working in a shared war reality. *British Journal of Social Work*, 39(6), 1154-1174.

Levine, P. (2005). *Healing trauma: a pioneering program for restoring the wisdom of your body*. Boulder CO: Sounds True.

Levy, H.C., Conoscenti, L.M., Tillery, J.F., Dickstein, B.D. & Litz, B.T. (2011). Deployment stressors and outcomes among Air Force chaplains. *Journal of Traumatic Stress*, 24(3), 342-346.

Lewis, C.A., Turton, D.W. & Francis, L.J. (2007). Clergy work-related psychological health, stress and burnout: an introduction to this special issue of Mental Health, Religion and Culture. *Mental Health, Religion & Culture*, 10(1), 1-8.

Lombardo, K.L., & Motta, R.W. (2008). Secondary trauma in children of parents with mental illness. *Traumatology*, 14(3), 57-67.

Lount, M. & Hargie, O. (1997). The priest as counselor: an investigation of critical incidents in the pastoral work of Catholic priests. *Counselling Psychology Quarterly*, 10(3), 246-258.

Lount, M. and Hargie, O. (1998). Preparation for the priesthood: a training needs analysis. *Journal of Vocational Education and Training*, 50(1), 61-77.

Lucas, L. (2008). The Pain of Attachment "you have to put a little wedge in there": how vicarious trauma affects child/teacher attachment. *Childhood Education*, 84(2), 85-90.

Ludick, M., & Figley, C. R. (2017). Toward a mechanism for secondary trauma induction and reduction: Reimagining a theory of secondary traumatic stress. *Traumatology*, 23(1), 112-123.

Lyon, E. (1993). Hospital staff reactions to accounts by survivors of childhood abuse. *American Journal of Orthopsychiatry*, 63, 410-416.

McAllister, R.J. (1993). Mental health treatment of religious professionals. In R.J. Wicks & D. Capps (Eds.), *Clinical handbook of pastoral counseling, 2*, (pp. 208-227). Mahwah NJ: Paulist Press.

McAloney, K., McCrystal, P., Percy, A. & McCartan, C. (2009). Damaged youth: prevelance of community violence exposure and implications for adolscent well-being in post-conflict Northern Ireland. *Journal of Community Psychology*, 37(5), 653-648.

McBride, B.E. (2007). Prevalence of secondary traumatic stress among social workers. *Social Work*, 52, 63-70.

McCaffrey, T. (2004). Responding to Crises in Schools: A consultancy model for supporting schools in Crisis. *Educational & Child Psychology* 2004, 21(3), 109-120.

McCann, I.L. & Pearlman, L.A. (1990a). *Psychological trauma and the adult survivor: theory, therapy and transformation*. New York: Brummer/Mazel.

McCann, I.L. & Pearlman, L.A. (1990b). Vicarious traumatization: a framework for understanding the effects of trauma on helpers. *Journal of Traumatic Stress*, 3 (1), 131-149.

McCann, I.L. & Pearlman, L.A. (1990c). *Through a looking glass darkly: understanding and treating the adult trauma survivor through Constructivist Self Development Theory*. New York: Brunner/Mazel.

McCann, I.L. & Saakvitne, K.W. (1995). Treating therapists with vicarious traumatization and secondary traumatic stress disorders. In C.R. Figley (Ed.), *Compassion fatigue: Coping with secondary traumatic stress disorder in those who treat the traumatized* (pp.150-177). New York: Brunner/Mazel.

McLaughlin, C. (2008). Emotional wellbeing and its relationship to schools and classrooms: a critical reflection. *British Journal of Guidance & Counselling*, 36(4), 352-366.

McLeod, J. (2003). *An introduction to counselling*. 3rd Ed. Maidenhead: Open University Press.

McMinn, M.R., Lish, A., Trice, P.D., Root, A.M., Gilbert, N. & Yap, A. (2005). Care for pastors: learning from clergy and their spouses. *Pastoral Psychology*, 53(6), 563-581.

MacRitchie, V. & Leibowitz, S. (2010). Secondary traumatic stress, level of exposure, empathy and social support in trauma workers. *South African Journal of Psychology*, 40, 149-158.

Mannon, D. & Crawford, R. (1996). Clergy confidence to counsel and their willingness to refer to mental health professionals. *Family Therapy*, 23, 213-231.

Marmar, C., Weiss, D., Metzler, T. & Delucchi, K. (1996). Characteristics of emergency services personnel related to peritraumatic dissociation during critical incident exposure. *American Journal of Psychiatry*, 153(supp), 94-102.

Maslach, C. (1976). Burned-out. *Human Behavior*, 5, 16-22.

Maslach, C. & Jackson, S.E. (1986). *Maslach Burnout Inventory manual*. (2nd Ed). Palo Alto, CA: Consulting Psychological Press

Maslach, C., Schaufeil, W. & Leiter, M. (2001). Job Burnout. *Annual Review Psychology*, 52, 397-422.

Mathews, M. (2007). An investigation of Singaporean clergy treatment models for mental problems. *Journal of Religious Health*, 46, 558-570.

Matthews, G., Zeidner, M. & Roberts, R. (2004). *Emotional Intelligence: science and myth*. Cambridge, MA: MIT Press.

Mayer, J.D. & Salovey, P. (1997). What is emotional intelligence? In P. Salovey & D. Sluyter (Eds.) Emotional development and emotional ability. *Educational Implications*, (pp. 3-31). New York: Basic Books.

Maytum, J.C., Heiman, M.B. & Garwick, A.W. (2004). Compassion fatigue and burnout in nurses who work with children with chronic conditions and their families. *Journal of Paediatric Health Care*, 18(4), 171-179.

Maxwell, J.A. (2005). *Qualitative research design*. Thousand Oaks, CA: Sage.

Meek, K.R., McMinn, M.R., Brower, C.M., Burnett, T.D., McRay, B.W., Ramey, M.L., Swanson, D.W., & Villa, D.D. (2003). Maintaining personal resiliency: Lessons learned from evangelical protestant clergy. *Journal of Psychology and Theology*, 31, 339-347.

Meldrum, L., King, R., & Spooner, D. (2002). Secondary traumatic stress in case managers working in community mental health services. Figley, Charles R (Ed.). *Treating compassion fatigue*, (pp. 85-106) New York: New York: Brunner Routledge.

Merriam Webster. (2009). Merriam Webster On-line Dictionary. Available from http://www.merriam-webster.com/dictionary/trauma [Accessed 1 Nov 2009].

Meyers, T.W. & Cornille, T.A. (2002). The work of working with traumatized children. In C.R. Figley (Ed.). *Treating compassion fatigue*. New York: Brunner/Mazel.

Miles, M.B. & Huberman, A.M. (1994). *Qualitative data analysis: an expanded sourcebook*. Thousand Oaks, CA: Sage.

Miner, J.B. (1992). *Industrial Organisational Psychology*. New York: McGraw-Hill

Miner, M.A. (2007a). Changes in burnout over the first 12 months in ministry: links with stress and orientation. *Mental Health, Religion & Culture*, 10(1), 9-16.

Miner, M.A. (2007b), Burnout in the first years of ministry: personality and belief style as important predictors. Mental Health, Religion & Culture, 10(1), 17-29.

Mollica, R.F. (1988). The trauma Story: the psychiatric care of refugee survivors of violence and torture. In F.M. Ochberg (Ed.) *Posttraumatic Therapy and Victims of Violence* (pp. 295-314). New York: Brunner/Mazel.

Morgan, H. (2004). Spiritual healing. *Learning Disability Practice, 7*(5), 8-9.

Morrison, T. (2007). Emotional Intelligence, emotion and social work: context, characteristics, complications and contribution. *The British Journal of Social Work, 37*(2), 245-263.

Motta, R.W. (2008). Secondary trauma. *International Journal of Emergency Mental Health, 10*(4), 291-298.

Motta, R.W., Joseph, J., Rose, R., Suszzi, J. & Leiderman, l. (1997). Secondary trauma: assessing intergenerational transmission of war experiences with a modified stroop procedure. *Journal of Clinical Psychology, 53*, 895-903.

Munroe, J.F. (1999). Ethical issues associated with secondary trauma in therapists. In B.H. Stamm, (Ed.) *Secondary Traumatic Stress. Self-Care Issues for Clinicians, Researchers and Educators.* (2nd Ed.). Baltimore: Sidran Press

Murphy-Geiss, G.E. (2011). Married to the Minister: The Status of the Clergy Spouse as Part of a Two-Person Single Career. *Journal of Family Issues, 32*(7), 932–955.

Najjar, N., Davis, L.W., Beck-Coon, K. & Doebbeling, C.C. (2009). Compassion fatigue: a review of the research to date and the relevance to cancer care providers. *Journal of Health Psychology, 14*(2), 267-277.

Neergaard, J.A., Lee, J.W., Anderson, B. & Gengler, S.W. (2007). Women experiencing intimate partner violence: effects of confiding in religious leaders. *Pastoral Psychology, 55*(6), 773-787.

Neff, K.D. (2003). Self–compassion: an alternative conceptualization of a health attitude towards oneself. *Self & Identity, 2*, 85-102.

Nolen-Hoeksema, S. (1991). Responses to depression and their effects on the duration of depressive episodes. *Journal of Abnormal Psychology, 100*, 569–582.

Nolen-Hoeksema, S., Wisco, B.E. & Lyubomirsky, S. (2008). Rethinking rumination. *Perspectives on Psychological Science, 3*(5), 400-424.

O'Kane, S. & Millar, R. (2001). An investigation into the counselling-type work of Roman Catholic priests: a survey of one diocese in Northern Ireland. *British Journal of Guidance & Counselling, 29* (3). 323-335.

O'Kane, S. & Millar, R. (2002). A qualitative study of pastoral counselling of Catholic priests in one diocese in Northern Ireland. *British Journal of Guidance & Counselling, 30*(2), 189-206.

Oman, D. & Thoresen, C.E. (2005). Do religion and spirituality influence health. In R.F. Paloutzian & C.L. Clark (Eds.) *Handbook of the psychology of religion and spirituality*, (pp. 435-459). New York: Guilford Press.

Oppenheimer, J.E., Julia, E., Kevin, J., Flannelly, A. & Weaver, A. (2004). Comparative analysis of the psychological literature on collaboration between clergy and mental-health professionals-perspectives from secular and religious journals:1970-1999. *Pastoral Psychology, 53*, 153-162.

Ortlepp, K. & Friedman, M. (2002). Prevalence and correlates of secondary traumatic stress in workplace lay trauma counselors. *Journal of Traumatic Stress, 15*, 213-222.

Oswald, R. M. (1991). *Clergy self-care: Finding a balance for effective ministry.* New York: The Alban Institute, Inc.

Parker, J.D.A., Taylor, G. J., & Bagby, R. M. (2001). The relationship between emotional intelligence and alexithymia. *Personality and Individual Differences, 30*, 107-115.

Pau, A.K.H. & Croucher, R. (2003). Emotional Intelligence and perceived stress in dental undergraduates. *Journal of Dental Education, 67*, 1023-1028.

Pearlman, L.A. (1995). Self-care for trauma therapists. Ameliorating vicarious traumatization. In B.H. Stamm (Ed.) *Secondary traumatic stress: self-care issues for clinicians, researchers and educators (*pp. 51-64). Lutherville, MD: Sidran.

Pearlman, L.A. (2003). *Trauma and Attachment Belief Scale: manual.* Los Angles CA: Western Psychological Services.

Pearlman, L.A. & Mac Ian, P.S. (1993). Vicarious traumatization amongst trauma therapists: empirical findings on self-care. Trauma Stress Points: *News for the International Society for Traumatic Stress studies, 7*(3), 5.

Pearlman, L.A. & Mac Ian, P.S. (1995). Vicarious traumatization: An empirical study of the effects of trauma work on trauma therapists. *Professional Psychology: Research Practice*, 26(6), 558-565.

Pearlman, L.A. & McKay, L. (2008). *Understanding and coping with vicarious trauma: on-line training module.* Pasadena, CA: Headington Institute.

Pearlman, L.A. & Saakvitne, K.W. (1995a). Treating therapists with vicarious traumatization and secondary traumatic stress disorders. In C.R. Figley (Ed.) *Compassion fatigue: coping with secondary traumatic stress disorder in those who treat the traumatized.* (pp.150-177). Levittown, PA: Brunner/Mazel.

Pearlman, L.A. & Saakvitne, K.W. (1995b). Constructivist self-development theory and trauma therapy. Pearlman, L.A. & Saakvitne, K.W. (Ed.) *Trauma and the therapist: countertransference and vicarious traumatization in psychotherapy with incest survivors*, (pp. 55-74) New York: New York: Norton.

Pearlman, L. A. & Saakvitne, K.W. (1995c). *Trauma and the therapist: countertransference and vicarious traumatization in psychotherapy with incest survivors.* New York: Norton.

Pennebaker, J.W. (1997). *Opening Up: The Healing Power of Expressing Emotions* (Revised edition). New York: Guilford Press.

Perry, B., Toffner, G., Merrick, T. & Dalton, J. (2011). An exploration of the experience of compassion fatigue in clinical oncology nurses. *Canadian Oncology Nursing Journal*, 21(2), 91-105.

Petrides, K.V. & Furnham, A. (2003). Trait Emotional Intelligence: behavioural validation into studies of emotional recognition and reactivity to mood induction. *European Journal of Personality*, 17, 39-57.

Pfeil, S.M. (2006). A new understanding of clergy compassion fatigue for facilitators of trainings for the prevention of sexual misconduct. *Journal of Religion & Abuse.* 8(3), 63-78.

Phelps, A., Lloyd, D., Creamer, M. & Forbes, D. (2009). Caring for the carers in the aftermath of trauma. *Journal of Aggression, maltreatment & trauma,*18, 312-330

Piaget, J. (1971). *Psychology and epistemology: towards a theory of knowledge.* New York: Viking.

Price, M. (2001). *Secondary traumatization: vulnerability factors for mental health professionals.* Unpublished doctoral dissertation. University of Texas.

Quinal, L., Harford, S., & Rutledge, D.N. (2009). Secondary traumatic stress in oncology staff. *Cancer Nursing*, 32, 1-7.

Quinley, H. E. (1974). *The Prophetic Clergy: Social Activism Among Protestant Ministers.* New York: Wiley.

Radey, M. & Figley, C.R. (2007). The social psychology of compassion. *Clinical Social Work Journal,* 35(3), 207-214.

Raj, A. & Dean. K.E. (2005). Burnout and depression among Catholic priests in India. *Pastoral Psychology,* 54, 157-171.

Ramos, N.S., Fernandez-Berrocal, P. & Extremera, N. (2007). Perceived emotional intelligence facilitates cognitive-emotional processes of adaption to acute stressor. *Cognition & Emotion,* 21(4), 758-772.

Randall, K.J. (2004). Burnout as a Predictor of Leaving Anglican Parish Ministry. *Review of Religious Research*, 46(1), 20-26.

Randall, K.J. (2007). Examining the relationship between burnout and age among Anglican clergy in England and Wales. *Mental Health, Religion & Culture, 10(1), 39-46.*

Rayburn, C.A., Richmond, L.J. & Rogers, L. (1986). Men, women and religion: stress within leadership roles. *Journal of Clinical Psychology*, 42, 540-546.

Regehr, C. (2005). Bringing home the trauma: Spouses of paramedics. *Journal of Loss and Trauma,* 10(2), 97-114.

Regehr, C., Goldberg, G. & Hughes, J. (2002). Exposure to human tragedy, empathy and trauma in ambulance paramedics. *American Journal of Orthopsychiatry,* 72(4), 505-513.

Resick, P. (2000). *Stress and trauma.* Psychology Press: Hove.

Riley, H. & Schutte, N.S. (2003). Low Emotional Intelligence as a predictor for substance-use problems. *Journal of Drug Education*, 33(4), 391-398

Robbins, P.M., Meltzer, L. & Zelikovsky, N. (2009). The experience of secondary traumatic stress upon care providers working within a children's hospital. *Journal of Pediatric Nursing*, 24(4), 270-279.

Roberts, S.B., Flannelly, K.J., Weaver, A.J. & Figley, C.R. (2003). Compassion fatigue among chaplins, clergy, and other respondants after September 11th. *The Journal of Nervous and Mental Diseases*, 191(11), 756-758.

Rodgerson, T.E. & Piedmont, L. (1998). Assessing the incremental validity of Religious Problem-Solving Scale in the prediction of clergy burnout. *Journal for the Scientific Study of Religion*, 37, 517-527.

Rogers, C.R. (1951). *Client-centered Therapy: Its Current Practice, Implications and Theory*. London: Constable.

Rothschild, B. & Rand, M.L. (2006). *Help for the helper: the psychophysiology of compassion fatigue and vicarious trauma*. NewYork: Norton.

Rudolfsson, L. & Tidefors, I. (2009). "Shepherd my sheep"; clerical readiness to meet psychological and existential needs from victims of sexual abuse. *Pastoral Psychology*, 58, 79-92.

Rudolph, J.M. & Stamm, B.H. (1999). Maximising Human Capital: Moderating Secondary Traumatic Stress through Administrative & Policy Action. In B.H. Stamm, (Ed.) *Secondary Traumatic Stress. Self-Care Issues for Clinicians, Researchers and Educators. (2nd Ed.)*. Baltimore: Sidran Press.

Russell, A. (1984). *A clerical profession*. London: SPCK.

Rutledge, C.J.F. & Francis, L.J. (2004). Burnout among male Anglican parochial clergy in England: testing a modified form of the Maslach Burnout Inventory. *Research in the Social Scientific Study of Religion*, 15, 71-93.

Saakvitne, K. & Pearlman, L. (1996). *Transforming the pain: A workbook on vicarious traumatization*. W.W. Norton & Co.

Sabin-Farrell, R. & Turpin, G. (2003). Vicarious traumatization: implications for the mental health of health workers? *Clinical Psychology Review*, 23(3), 449-480.

Sabo, B.M. (2006). Compassion fatigue and nursing work: can we accurately capture the consequences of caring work? *International Journal of Nursing Practice*, 12(3), 136-142.

Salovey, P., Bedell, B., Detweiler, J.B. & Mayer, J. (1999). Coping intelligently: Emotional intelligence and the coping process. In C.R. Snyder (Ed.) *Coping: the psychology of what works* (pp. 141-164). New York: Oxford University Press.

Salovey, P. & Mayer, J.D. (1990). Emotional Intelligence. *Imagination, Cognition & Personality*, 9, 185-211.

Salovey, P., Woolery, A., Stroud, L. & Epel, E. (2002). Perceived emotional intelligence, stress reactivity and symptoms reports: further explorations using The Trait Meta-Mood Scale. *Psychology & Health*, 17, 611-627.

Salston, M. & Figley, C.R. (2003). Secondary traumatic stress effects of working with survivors of criminal victimization. *Journal of Traumatic Stress*, 16, 167-174.

Sanford, J. (1982). *Ministry burnout*. London: Arthur James Ltd.

Scaturo, D.J. & Hayman, P.M. (1992). The impact of combat trauma across family life cycles: clinical considerations. *Journal of Traumatic Stress*, 5(2), 273-288.

Schauben, L.J. & Frazier, P.A. (1995). Vicarious trauma: the effects on female counselors of working with sexual violence survivors. *Psychological Woman*, 19, 49-64.

Schulster, M.A., Stein, B.D., Jaycox, L.H., Collins, R.L., Marshall, G.N., Elliott, M.N., Zhou, A.J., Kanouse, D.E., Morrison, J.L. & Berry, S.H. (2001). A national survey of stress reactions after the September 11, 2001 terrorist attacks. *New England Journal of Medicine*, 345(20), 1507-1512.

Schutte, N.S., Malouff, J.M., Bobik, C., Coston, T.D., Greeson, C., Jedlicka, C., Rhodes, E. & Wendorf, G. (2001). Emotional Intelligence and interpersonal relations. The *Journal of Social Psychology*, 141(4), 523-536.

Sexton, L. (1999). Vicarious traumatisation of counsellor and effects on their workplace. *British Journal of Guidance & Counselling*, 27(3), 393-403.

Shah, S.A., Garland, E. & Katz, C. (2007). Secondary traumatic stress: prevalence in humanitarian aid workers in India. *Traumatology*, 13(1), 59-70.

Sherman, A.C., Edwards, D., Simonton, S. & Mehta, P. (2006). Caregiver stress and burnout in an oncology unit. *Palliative & Support Care*, 4(1), 65-80.

Shulman, L. (1990). *The skills of helping: individuals and groups*. Illinois: Peacock.

Sibert, D.C. (2004). Depression in North Carolina social workers: Implications for practice and research. *Social Work Research*, 28, 30-40.

Siegel, K., Anderman, S.J. & Schrimshaw, E.W. (2001). Religion and coping with health-related stress. *Psychology & Health*, 16(6), 631-653.

Sifneos, P.E. (1972). *Short term psychotherapy and emotional crisis*. Cambridge, MA: Harvard University Press.

Sigmund, J.A. (2003). Spirituality and trauma: the role of clergy in the treatment of Posttraumatic Stress Disorder. *Journal of Religion & Health*, 42(3), 221-229.

Simon, C., Pryce, J., Roff, L. & Klemmack, D. (2005). Secondary traumatic stress and oncology social work: protecting compassion from fatigue and compromising the workers worldview. *Journal of Psychological Oncology*, 23(4), 1-14.

Simonds, S.L. (1996). *Vicarious traumatization in therapists treating adult survivors of childhood sexual abuse*. Unpublished doctoral dissertation. The Fielding Institute.

Sinclair, H.A.H. & Hamill, C. (2007). Does vicarious traumatisation affect oncology nurses? A literature review. *European Journal of Oncology Nursing*, 11(4), 348-356.

Slaski, M. & Cartwright, S. (2002). Health performance and emotional intelligence: an exploratory study of retail managers. *Stress & Health*, 18, 63-68.

Slattery, S. & Goodman, L.A. (2009). Secondary traumatic stress among domestic violence advocates: workplace risk and protective factors. *Violence Against Women*, 15(11), 1358-1379.

Sluka, J.A. (2009). In the shadows of the gun. *Critique of Anthropology*, 29(3), 279-299.

Smith, D.P. & Orlinsky, D.E. (2004). Religious and spiritual experience among psychotherapist. *Psychotherapy: Theory, research, practice & training*, 41(2), 144-151.

Smith, J. (2004). Reexamining Psychotherapeutic Action Through the Lens of Trauma. *Journal of American Academy of Psychoanalysis*, 32, 613-631.

Smollan, R. & Parry, K. (2011). Follower perception of the emotional intelligence of change leaders: a qualitative study. *Leadership*, 7(4), 435-462.

Sommer, C.A. (2008). Vicarious traumatization: trauma-sensitive supervision and counselor preparation. *Counsellor Education and Supervision*, 48(1), 61-71.

Spencer, J.L., Winston, B.E. & Bocarnea, M.C. (2012). Predicting the Level of Pastors' Risk of Termination/Exit from the Church. *Pastoral Psychology*,61(1), 85-98.

Sprang, G., Clark, J.J. & Whitt-Woosley, A. (2007). Compassion fatigue, compassion satisfaction and burnout: factors impacting a professional's quality of life. *Journal of Loss & Trauma, 12, 259-280.*

Stamm, B.H. (1999*). Secondary traumatic stress: Self-care issues for clinicians, researchers and educators*. 2nd ed. Maryland: Sidran Press: Lutherville.

Stamm, B.H. (2002). Measuring compassion satisfaction as well as fatigue: Developmental history of the compassion satisfaction and fatigue test. Figley, C.R. (Ed.) *Treating compassion fatigue*, (pp. 107-119) New York: Brunner/Routledge.

Stamm, B.H. (2002). *The ProQOL Manua III: The Professional Quality of Life Scale: Compassion Satisfaction, Burnout & Compassion Fatigue/Secondary Trauma Scales*. Baltimore, MD: Sidra Press

Stamm, B.H. (2005). *The ProQOL Manual IV: The Professional Quality of Life Scale: Compassion Satisfaction, Burnout & Compassion Fatigue/Secondary Trauma Scales*. Baltimore, MD: Sidra Press.

Stamm, B.H. (2009). *The concise ProQOL V Manual*. Baltimore, MD: Sidran Press.Available from http://compassionfatigue.org/pages/ProQOLManual [Accessed 20 November 2009].

Stanford, M.S. & McAlister, K.R. (2008). Perceptions of serious mental illness in the local church. *Journal of Religion, Disability & Health*, 12(2), 144-153.

Stanton, A.L., Danoff-Burg, S., Cameron, C.L., Bishop, M., Collins, C.A., Kirk, S.B., Sworowski, L.A. & Twillman, R. (2000). Emotionally expressive coping predicts psychological and physical adjustment to breast cancer. *Journal of Consulting & Clinical Psychology*, 68(5), 875-882.

Steed, L. & Dowling, R. (1998). A phenomenological study of vicarious traumatisation amongst psychologists and professional counselors working in the field of sexual abuse/assault. *Australasian Journal of Disaster and Trauma Studies*, 2, 1-8.

Suozzia, J.M. & Motta, R.A. (2004). The relationship between combat exposure and the transference of trauma like symptoms to offspring of veterans. *Traumatology*, 10(1), 17-37.

Switzer, D.K. (2000). *Pastoral care emergencies*. Minneapolis: Fortress Press.

Sy, T., Tram, S. & O'Hara, L.A. (2006). Relation of employee and manager emotional intelligence to job satisfaction and performance. *Journal of Vocational Behavior*, 68(3), 461-473.

Taylor, B.E., Flannelly, K.J., Weaver, A.J. & Zucker, D.J. (2006). Compassion fatigue and burnout among Rabbis working as chaplains. *The Journal of Care & Counseling*, 60(1-2), 35-41.

Tischler, L., Biberman, J. & McKeage, R. (2002). Linking emotional intelligence, spirituality and workplace performance: Definitions, models and ideas for research. *Journal of Managerial Psychology*, 17(3), 203-218.

Townsend, S.M. & Campbell, R. (2009). Organizational correlates of secondary traumatic stress and burnout among sexual assault nurse examiners, *Journal of Forensic Nursing*, 5, 97–106.

Traumatic Stress Institute, (1997). *Traumatic Stress Institute Belief Scale*. South Windsor, CT: Author.

Trinidad, D.R., Unger, J.B., Chou, C.P. & Johnson, C.A. (2004). The protective association between emotional intelligence with psychosocial smoking risk factors for adolescents. *Personality & Individual Differences*, 36, 945- 954.

Trippary, R.L. (2000). *Predictors of vicarious traumatisation: female therapists for adult survivors versus female therapists for child survivors of sexual victimization*. Unpublished doctoral dissertation. University of Alabama.

Trippany, R.L., White-Kress, V.E. & Wilcoxon, S.A. (2004). Preventing vicarious trauma: what counselors should know when working with trauma survivors. *Journal of Counseling & Development*, 82(1), 31-37.

Turton, D.W. (2010). *Clergy burnout and emotional exhaustion: a socio-psychological study of job stress and job satisfaction*. Lewiston: The Edwin Mellen Press.

Turton, D.W. & Francis, L.J. (2007). The relationship between attitude toward prayer and professional burnout among Anglican parochial clergy in England: Are praying clergy healthier clergy? *Mental Health, Religion and Culture, 10*, 61-74.

Vaillant, G. (2000). Adaptive mental mechanism: their role in a positive psychology. *American Psychologist*, 55(1), 89-98.

Van der Kolk, B.A. (1987). *Psychological Trauma*. Washington, DC: American Psychological Press.

Van der Kolk, B.A. & McFarlane, A.C. (1996). The black hole of trauma. In Van der Kolb, B.A., McFarlane, A.C. & Weisaeth, L. (Eds) *Traumatic stress: the effects of overwhelming experience on mind, body and society*. New York: Guilford Press.

Versola-Russo, J.M. (2007). Workplace violence: vicarious trauma in the psychiatric setting. *Journal of Police Crisis Negotiations*, 6(2), 79-103.

Virginia, S.G. (1998). Burnout and depression amongst Roman Catholic secular, religious and monastic clergy. *Pastoral Psychology*,47(1), 49-67.

Vrklevski, L.P. & Franklin, J. (2008). Vicarious trauma: the impact on solicitors of exposure to traumatic material. *Traumatology*, 14(1), 106-118.

Walker, M. (2001). The aftermath of abuse: the effects of counseling on the client and the counsellor. In P. Milner and S.E. Palmer (Eds.) *Counselling: the BACP counseling reader (*vol 2. pp. 246-252.). London: Sage Publications.

Walker, M. (2004). Supervising practitioners working with surviviors of childhood abuse: counter transference, secondary traumatization and terror. *Psychodynamic Practice: individuals, groups and organisations*, 10(2), 173-193.

Wang, P.S., Berglund, P.A. & Kessler, R.C. (2003). Patterns and correlates of contacting clergy for mental disorders in the United States. *Health Services Research, 38*(2), 647-673.

Warner, J. & Carter, J.D. (1984). Loneliness, martial adjustment and burnout in pastoral and lay persons. *Journal of Psychology and Theology*, 12, 125-131.

Wastell, C. (2002). Exposure to trauma: the cost of suppressing emotional reactions. *Journal of Nervous & Mental Disease*, 192, 849-857.

Way I., Van Deusen, K. & Cottrell, T. (2007). Vicarious trauma: Predictors of clinicians' disruptive conditions about self-esteem and self-intimacy. *Journal of Child Sexual Abuse,*16(4), 81-89.

Waysman, M., Mikulincer, M., Solomon, Z. & Weisenberg, M. (1993). Secondary traumatization among wives of posttraumatic combat veterans: A family typology. *Journal of Family Psychology*, 7, 104-118.

Weaks, K.A. (1999). *Effects of treating trauma survivors: vicarious trauma and style of coping*. Unpublished doctoral dissertation. Texas: Texas Woman's University.

Weaver, A.J. (1995). Has there been a failure to prepare and support parish-based clergy in their role as front-line community mental health workers? A review. *The Journal of Pastoral Care*, 49(2), 129-149.

Weaver, A.J., Flannelly, K.J., Flannelly, L.T. & Oppenheimer, J.E. (2003). Collaboration between clergy and mental health professionals: a review of professional heath care journals from 1980 through 1999. *Counseling & Values, 47,* 162-163.

Weaver, A.J., Koenig, F.M. & Ochberg, F.M. (1996). Posttraumatic stress. Mental health professionals, and the clergy: a need for collaboration, training and research. *Journal of Traumatic Stress,* 94(4), 847-856.

Wee, D. & Myers, D. (2002). Response of mental health workers following disaster. The Oklahoma City Bombing. In C.R. Figley (Ed.) *Treating compassion fatigue* (pp. 57-83). New York: Brunner/Rutledge.

Whetham, P. W., & Whetham, L. (2000). *Hard to be holy* Adelaide: Openbook.

White, G.D. (2001). Near ground zero: Compassion fatigue in the aftermath of September 11. *Traumatology*, 7(4), 151-154.

Wittine, B. (1995). The spiritual self: its relevance in the development and daily life of the psychotherapist. In M.B. Sussman (Ed.) *A perilous calling: the hazards of psychotherapy practice,* (pp288-301). New York: Wiley.

Wong, C.S. & Law, K.S. (2002). The effects of leader and follower Emotional Intelligence on performance and attitude: an exploratory study. *Leadership Quarterly*, 13, 243-274.

Wright, P.G. (1984). The counselling activities and referral practices of Canadian clergy in British Columbia. *Journal of Psychology & Theology*, 12(4), 294-304.

Ying, Y.W. (2009). Contribution of self-compassion to competence and mental health in social work students. *Journal of Social Work Education*, 45(2), 309-323.

Young, C.M. (1999). *Vicarious trauma in psychotherapists who work with physically or sexually abused children.* Unpublished doctoral dissertation. Alameda: The California School of Professional Psychology.

Young, J.L., Derr, D.M., Cicchillo, V.J. & Bressler, S. (2011). Compassion satisfaction burnout and secondary traumatic stress in heart and vascular nurses. *Critical Care Nursing Quarterly*, 3(3), 227-234.

Yule, W. (2000). Post-traumatic Stress Disorder in adults. In W. Yule (Ed.) *Post-Traumatic Stress Disorder: concepts and therapy.* 2nd Ed. Chichester: Wiley.